NOT JUST TALKING

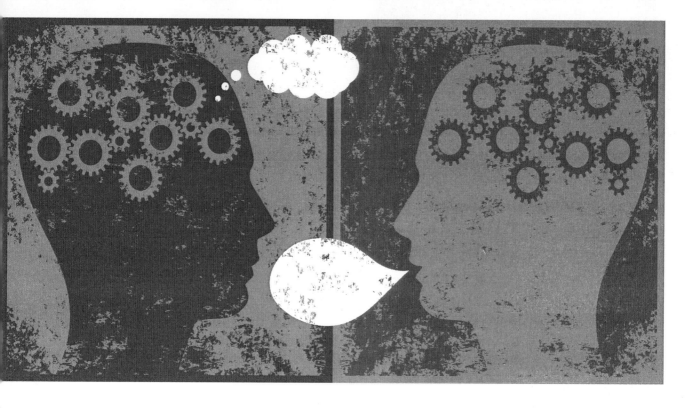

Identifying non-verbal communication difficulties - A life-changing approach

SIOBAN BOYCE

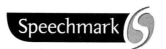

Published by
Speechmark Publishing Ltd, Sunningdale House, 43 Caldecotte Lake Drive, Milton Keynes
MK7 8LF, United Kngdom
Tel: +44 (0) 1908 277177
www.speechmark.net

002-5753/Printed in the United Kingdom by CMP (uk) Ltd

A catalogue record for this book is available from the British Library.

ISBN 978 086388849 6

CONTENTS

ACKNOWLEDGEMENTS

Many thanks to Hilary Whates for believing in my work and all her help in bringing this book to fruition and to Stephen for all the help he has given during its gestation!

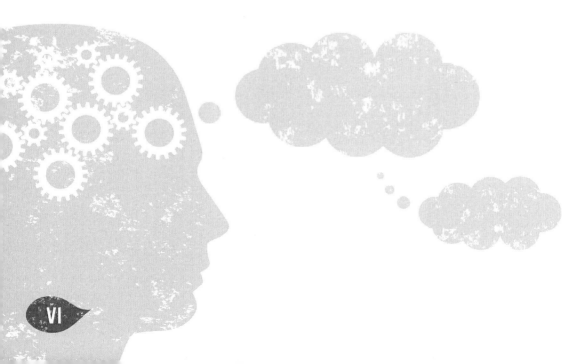

INTRODUCTION: TURNING THINGS AROUND

1

This book is about how the non-verbal communication skills that underpin our conversational ability are less likely to develop in the twenty-first century and the serious consequences for society of people growing up being able to talk but not to communicate. It introduces a new theory based on the skills children need to develop in the area of non-verbal communication. Widespread changes in society beginning in the last decades of the twentieth century mean that children have fewer opportunities to develop these essential communication skills.

The book begins by establishing the need for a new theory of communication development. It looks at research that supports this new theory and how it differs from current theories relating to child development. I then establish which skills we use as adults within a conversation that are the focus of this book and how central these skills are to our everyday life.

Section 3 looks at what has happened to change the way our children learn to communicate. There are then five sections covering the development of non-verbal communication skills from birth through to old age.

Once the 'normal' development has been explained, I look at the problems associated with failure to develop these non-verbal conversational skills. This is followed by an outline of the solutions I have developed, ranging from prevention through assessment to the Not Just Talking intervention techniques. This is followed by an outline of the training opportunities for all these three aspects of the solutions.

Conventions

Throughout this book I use 'he' and 'she' in different sections when referring to the child. Readers should assume that I am talking about matters that affect both boys and girls, unless I specify otherwise.

THE NOT JUST TALKING THEORY OF COMMUNICATION DEVELOPMENT

Current theories of the development of communication are predicated on language development. Most books, manuals and tests focus on the skills concerned with language comprehension and use. In education services for children with special needs it is understood that there are skills that precede language development, but even these programmes are based on attaining language development with a particular focus on speech.

Makaton, a signing programme that started in the 1970s, is an example of this. This programme made the assumption that the child needed to develop normal use of language and therefore the signs were introduced on this basis, establishing single noun use and then adding verbs, and so on.

The Intent to Communicate programme which was developed in the south of the UK in the late 1980s looked at what happened before the child began talking, and advocated steps that culminated in understanding and use of language skills, such as 'request action' and 'request object'.

In child development books for parents there is little about communication in the early months of the child's life, apart from information about babbling and listening skills. Again, this relates to language production and improving the chances of the baby learning to understand language.

This book hopes to show that language is actually an outcome of the development of non-verbal communication skills – none of which relate to language. If language starts, particularly spoken language, before these non-verbal skills develop sufficiently, then the child will learn to talk but may not be able to communicate effectively.

How this theory differs

This theory of communication development focuses on non-verbal communication skills, not verbal language. It shows how the development of non-verbal communication precedes, underpins and leads into the effective use of verbal language skills which we use to speak to one another.

In this book you will also discover why concentration on verbal language alone is no longer appropriate and can even be detrimental to the child's communication. The book aims to explain why children are growing up with so many communication problems nowadays and points to solutions which are cost-effective, simple, lasting and based on 15 years' successful experience of working in this way with children.

In the book I deal mainly with the development of essential non-verbal communication skills and what happens when they are lacking. These skills account for 60–90 per cent of how we understand the spoken message. As a by-product it is impossible not to mention the development of verbal communication occasionally, as this is a natural progression when good non-verbal skills are established.

Effective communication requires the development of a combination of many different skills that come together in the first five years of a child's life. The complex mix of elements related to language, such as grammar, vocabulary and articulation, is fully recognised. However, the non-verbal aspects of communication are by far the largest element. They are far-reaching and continue to mature over a lifetime. Verbal language development on the other hand reaches a peak by about the age of five years, and only the vocabulary develops after this as a person accumulates experiences where specific words are necessary.

Current understanding of non-verbal communication

In the late 1960s, ground-breaking research into communication and body language by Professor Albert Mehrabian (2007) found that in situations of confusion or inconsistency, 7 per cent of the message was conveyed by the words, 38 per cent by the voice and 55 per cent by the face. It was assumed by those interpreting his research that, by adding up the two figures, 93 per cent of communication was non-verbal at any one time. Since then, this interpretation has been discredited. The reason given is that the 38 per cent that Mehrabian attributed to the voice concerned spoken language and should not be added to the non-verbal side of the equation. But this way of interpreting Mehrabian's research demonstrates a lack of understanding of what constitutes the non-verbal element because it sees the 'voice' element that Mehrabian discussed – what is known as the prosodic element – as relating to verbal language development. This book will demonstrate how this 'vocal' element is in fact non-verbal because it refers to the way we change or add to the words using non-verbal features such as stress or intonation pattern.

Although Mehrabian's research was among the first to identify a dependence on facial expressions in particular to make good sense of complicated messages, what he didn't research was the effect of other non-verbal factors present in communication, which have more to do with the situation than what the person himself is conveying. In fact, his research focused only on how emotions are communicated through facial expressions and the like.

Being the only real research available on this specific point, my interpretation now shows that if we add body language and other supra-verbal communicating factors to the information given by the situation to aid comprehension of the verbal language, then the importance of non-verbal clues becomes even greater. By revisiting his percentages you will now see that at any one time, 60–90 per cent of communication is non-verbal – mostly relating to assisting comprehension of the spoken message.

Other views on the importance of non-verbal communication

Other writers have identified the importance of non-verbal understanding in adult life. Malcolm Gladwell (2005) has spoken to many researchers and writes about what he calls 'thin slicing' – the ability to process all the non-verbal information in the 'blink' of an eye and make a split-second judgements about what is going on. He reports that in adults this first interpretation is often the correct one, and we should be aware of its potential. Adults may change their minds after reflection, but later evidence often demonstrates that the first impression was accurate. My contention is that we also use this 'thin slicing' skill subconsciously to make moment-to-moment decisions about whether to say something, what to say, and how to say it. What Gladwell talks about is a very high-level skill that we develop in our teenage years, based on the development of the basic but essential non-verbal communication skills described in this book.

The experience that led to this new theory

Having trained as a speech and language therapist in the 1970s, I worked for nearly 20 years in the National Health Service. In the early 1980s children started entering my clinic, only one or two of them at first but many more by the end of the decade, whose verbal communication didn't seem to be a problem. These children were referred because their verbal understanding was slightly depressed, but it was difficult to tell from the standardised speech and language therapy assessments whether the child couldn't understand or was choosing not to answer (a significant problem associated with testing children with non-verbal difficulties, especially those on the autistic spectrum).

In the early 1990s, I was Head of Speech and Language Therapy for Learning Disabilities with a health authority. It was during this time that I became aware of the strong connection between challenging behaviour and communication problems. Since no one seemed to know the real reason why this was happening, I started looking at the research into what babies do in the early days of life. It was from this that I developed a new way of looking at communication and started to devise different ways of intervening with the children.

Speech and language models

The speech and language models applied in those days to the clients of learning disability services appeared to me to be a paediatric model based solely on speech and language development. The available assessments identified language problems: was the child or adult able to understand the information-carrying words and could they articulate and use vocabulary and grammar appropriately?

Based on this information, an intervention was planned to promote language use at the appropriate level towards the target of speech. Programmes devised would:

- improve auditory discrimination, memory or sequencing problems

- promote the production of sounds such as /b/, if the child was able to put his lips together, or other sounds

- help a child who couldn't understand colours or other adjectives to make sure he 'knew his colours', or the difference between 'big' and 'little', for example.

The fundamental problem experienced at that time, and it is probably still true 20 years later, was that this method of intervention improved skills in clinical settings, but the child found generalisation in the outside world difficult. This applied to all children, even those in mainstream schools.

By changing the emphasis to promoting only non-verbal communication skills, the Not Just Talking intervention programme's outcomes have generalisation at the centre. Once these skills are at the right level, language skills flow whatever the circumstances.

  Speechmark

The Not Just Talking vision

With regard to those people with a learning disability, whether verbal or not, applying this paediatric model appeared to be saying: 'We have a secret society called "language": we can all do it, so come and join us.' I asked myself some simple questions. Should those who can communicate try to get people with learning problems to pick up a new and complex skill of verbal language so that they can reach our level of communication and talk to us? Or was it easier for us, as good communicators, to start at the level of those with a learning disability and help them progress in simple steps from there?

This led to an end of the paediatric model in my department and the appearance of a model that valued the level of communication that had been achieved in each individual client, and then built their non-verbal skills from that point towards better communication. This vision is at the heart of all the methods of intervention and support used by Not Just Talking.

We made our communication as simple as the client needed so that he could understand what was being communicated. We made no assumptions about his level of understanding of language. Assumptions were also never made about what he was thinking, so reasons for his behaviour were not attributed, unless he could communicate what he was thinking for himself.

We used other methods of communication, such as objects, pictures, symbols, and so on, but always backed this up with help to develop facial interest and a sound understanding of what faces tell us, as well as all the other non-verbal clues described in this book. Situations were enhanced with obvious visual clues to act as pointers to the signals that tell us how to understand situations. The whole approach was to give support to the client to take control of his communication. When he no longer needed the supports, they were withdrawn and he progressed to the next level of communication.

Communicative settings

No client should be put in situations where carers are chatting away using language at high levels, which may include banter, if the client's communication and language skills are functioning below a five-year-old level. Children or adults with poor non-verbal understanding will not pick up language and communication skills just by listening. It will wash over them and may end up seriously confusing them. These essential non-verbal skills have to be developed first. The child's expressive language skills might well be commensurate with his age level, but if non-verbal skills lag behind, the same applies: he will not understand what is being said and will not learn simply by being exposed to conversations.

Another problem associated with pursuing a speech and language model of intervention is that the focus of the intervention is to promote the language skills of the child. If the child's non-verbal skills are far behind – 14-year-olds can be functioning at a pre-three-year level with regard to non-verbal communication – all language intervention does is develop his language skills. The consequence of this is that the gap between his good expressive language skills and his poor conversational skills just gets bigger.

WHY A NEW MODEL IS NEEDED

The speech and language model of communication development is not the only model to fail to address non-verbal communication. Other forms of support and therapy for children are commonly planned on a similar basis.

Psychotherapeutic model

Midwives tend to focus on establishing bonding between babies and parents based on a psychotherapeutic model of communication which sees bonding as the first step in the interaction between parents and their new baby. This is based on developing a loving relationship with your baby. This loving relationship is believed to promote care and attention from parent to child and hence the well-being of the infant.

After reading this book, you will understand how, before bonding can happen, the baby needs to develop non-verbal communication skills. It is these fundamental skills that enable bonding to take place. Many parents struggle to bond with babies. However, the Not Just Talking approach takes the blame away from the baby and the parent and gives parents something functional to work on. This is something which takes place between parent and child without the emphasis on success or failure to bond. The approach is also fun and shows almost immediate progress. Bonding will happen as a consequence of the parents interacting with their baby to promote facial interest and the give-and-take of conversations.

Psychological model

Although this model works well with children who don't suffer from communication difficulties, it is problematic for children with poor non-verbal understanding for two main reasons:

1 Most current strategies are based on language and thought development – both of which are dependent on the development of non-verbal communication skills. So the same applies as for the speech and language models: these skills will be promoted to the detriment of the conversational skills.

2 Intervention and strategies used when working with people with learning disability or on the autistic spectrum are based on behaviourist principles.

The behaviourist approach can be described simplistically as: when the child achieves the target behaviour he receives a reward. In my view this is an unrealistic approach to communication because it doesn't take account of the complexity of non-verbal or verbal communication or the need to develop understanding.

The behaviourist approach doesn't teach the child how to recognise the signals for applying the behaviour which is essential if he is to reproduce it at will. This sets the child up for failure as adults think that he has been supported to produce the behaviour appropriately. Because the child is not taught how to recognise the non-verbal signals, children with learning disability and on the autistic spectrum frequently appear to be unable to generalise their learning. You will understand when you have read this book that generalisation is one of the main outcomes of the Not Just Talking intervention and prevention programmes.

The other problem with using behaviourist strategies is that often the targets set are too complex for the communication skill level of the child.

Educational model

The educational model has many elements to it – speech and language development, behaviourist strategies and teaching models. It is this last element that I shall discuss here, particularly with reference to primary teaching.

Most teaching that I've observed has been based on the principle that if you can 'befriend' a child then you can get them to do what you want, ie, listen and learn. However, as teachers will be aware, particularly at secondary level, because of the poor development of conversational skills, children's behaviour nowadays is much less 'biddable' and therefore more of a battle for teachers. Without these essential non-verbal communication skills, children can't hold effective conversations. If a child can't hold a conversation then he can't make friends – with teachers or anyone else. So if you base your work with children on befriending them, you will struggle to be successful. This book will show how to promote these skills so that this model of successful teaching can be allowed to work.

WHAT IS NON-VERBAL COMMUNICATION?

The high percentage of non-verbal understanding conveyed in any communication comprises much more than understanding facial expressions and body language. The signals necessary to make good sense of the spoken message include:

1 facial expressions

2 body language

3 situational signals – location, surroundings, context, time, other people, etc

4 experiential information – previous experience of comparable circumstances

5 cognitive skills with regard to drawing conclusions, anticipation and prediction

6 plus all the prosodic information conveyed by intonation, volume, stress, rhythm and rate.

My view is that although the situational clues are the greatest in number, body language and facial expression are the most complex (these are treated separately in this book because they can communicate different things at the same time).

The origins of non-verbal communication problems

Non-verbal communication normally develops before a baby begins to talk and continues to develop alongside verbal language as the child becomes an increasingly proficient speaker. We are not born with these skills, but until about 1980 they developed naturally and nobody even thought much about them. Nowadays children have to work hard to acquire non-verbal understanding and avoid the risk of a life of social isolation and confusion.

Since the widespread use of the buggy which replaced the parent-facing pushchair in the 1980s, and which began to limit a child's scope to observe conversations in full flow, a great many other changes to the way we live our lives and how we communicate with one another have taken place. Now, in the second decade of twenty-first century, opportunities for children to absorb non-verbal skills are continually reduced, not least because we appear to hold fewer face-to-face conversations per day than we used to.

The family meal table – traditionally a key place for babies and children to observe and learn to understand the essential non-verbal aspects of conversations – is one situation where conversation has diminished significantly in the past 30 years. Whereas in the 1960s, when I grew up, we had three meals a day round the table, either at home or at school, now it is commonplace for children to eat alone or in front of the TV.

Recently I asked a group of approximately 150 people who were education workers – teachers, advisers, and so on – how many of them ate one meal a week round the table without a TV on. About 30–40 per cent put their hands up.

I then asked how many of them did this three times a day and no one put their hand up. This is just one of the major changes to our society that diminishes the number of opportunities for babies and children to observe and learn to understand the essential non-verbal component of conversations.

Is a new profession needed?

Because this is such a new approach to communication and completely different from the speech and language approach, I am of the view that perhaps a new profession should be developed. Speech and language therapists are excellent at working on language skills, but they are not the only people who can undertake the Not Just Talking intervention. I have successfully trained support workers, teachers, social workers, and so on, and also one or two speech and language therapists. The difficulty for speech and language therapists is that in order to do the therapy, you need to let go of what you know and feel about language development. If you view the child in the conventional way you will not be able to be as effective with the intervention.

Also, in relation to supervision, those professions with a language or a behaviourist background would be less conducive to serving this function. The Not Just Talking technique is much more akin to the disciplines of philosophy and sociology and so a new profession might use principles similar to those.

THE NOT JUST TALKING INTERVENTION

My early attempts achieved more success than intervention centred on speech and language alone, and encouraged me to develop a distinctive programme of non-verbal communication assessment and intervention. This comprised:

1 a simple but effective assessment giving a clear analysis of all the communication skills of the child, including non-verbal and verbal skills, within a half-hour session

2 an intervention method that, within six weeks of half-hour sessions, improves the child's communication, giving:

- complete generalisation of the skills learned

- theory of mind

- good information-giving appropriate to the context

- improved socialisation

- emotional understanding and communication

- improved understanding of spoken language

- improvements in grammar and other language difficulties

- an inability to return to the previous state of communication confusion

- improved auditory memory and sequencing skills

- the ability to progress academically.

See Section 12 for more about the intervention.

A note on differences between boys and girls

It's a commonly held view that boys find it harder to learn how to hold conversations and therefore are slower to develop language – but they get there in the end!

Until recently no one really knew why this occurred. It was just 'one of those things'. It was a 'given' and nobody in the speech and language therapy world appeared to question it. But towards the end of the twentieth century it was discovered that there is a big difference between the male and the female brain. The corpus callosum (the neural fibres which connect the left and right hemispheres) is larger in women, and this has significant repercussions for communication. A larger area with more neural pathways means that messages travel much faster between the two hemispheres of the brain. Therefore the language centre (Broca's area) on the left side of the brain can communicate with the right hemisphere, where interpretation of non-verbal information mainly occurs.

Simon Baron-Cohen (2003), a leading researcher into problems associated with autism, doesn't commit himself to whether this demonstrates a link between the better communication and empathy in women. This may be because the research he investigated was looking for better language skills rather than non-verbal skills. Baron-Cohen reports that women who had larger splenial areas (the rounded posterior area) in the corpus callosum did better on tests of verbal fluency.

Baron-Cohen reports the excitement generated by research that demonstrated a difference in the processing areas in the brain used for language tasks. Women use both sides of their brains but for men, language processing was only found in the left hemisphere. Remember that the hemisphere dominance tends to change if the man or woman is left-handed – the right hemisphere becomes dominant for language processing and execution.

My interpretation of this research is that possibly there is not another language area in women, it is just that the non-verbal processing area is able to communicate directly and at speed with the language centre in Broca's area on the opposite side of the brain, enabling the language area to access the non-verbal elements of communication.

So what has all this got to do with boys learning to hold conversations? The slower pace of development in boys was less evident when there were more opportunities (and more time) for them to acquire non-verbal skills. But in my view, it is likely that the physical make-up of the male brain means that boys will struggle more than girls to compensate for the lack of opportunity to acquire non-verbal understanding and skill. This would account for the fact that until relatively recently my caseload was 99 per cent male.

However, girls are now showing increased evidence of non-verbal difficulties. When I stopped working regularly with children in 2010 the proportion of boys in my caseload had dropped to less than 80 per cent. I believe this is due to two related factors:

1   The generation of children born in the 1980s when the development of non-verbal skills began to diminish have now grown up and have families of their own.

2   If you haven't developed these skills sufficiently yourself it is likely that you won't promote them in your children.

Therefore the problem gets worse in each generation, and the opportunities to observe effective conversations diminish further.

Mental health implications

I am fairly certain that non-verbal interpretational problems play a big part in conditions such as paranoia and schizophrenia. I know that in children these communication problems cause depression, thinking that they are hearing voices in their heads, anxiety, isolation, and so on, but this is not an area I have moved into because of the constant demand within mainstream and learning disability services. However, this could be a fruitful area of research.

It is possible to imagine that people with mental health problems could improve because they would be able to communicate better and participate effectively in counselling therapies if their non-verbal skills were addressed. I have witnessed demonstrable change in Asperger's and autistic children I have worked with who, although still on the spectrum, can communicate their feelings and difficulties to those around them in appropriate ways.

SO WHY THIS BOOK?

My fear is that if nothing is done to change the current pattern, the skills will continue to diminish with each subsequent generation. The potential social cost of this in terms of poor educational attainment, family breakdown, anti-social behaviour, criminality and so forth could be huge.

Yet the techniques I advocate are very simple and straightforward. What's more, they can unlock the child's potential, enabling him to communicate in whatever situation he finds himself. And this is the key to so much that is fulfilling, especially in learning and relationships. I hope that by the end of this book you will share my conviction that the development of effective non-verbal skills can change children's lives for the better. The Not Just Talking Intervention Resource Pack (planned for publication in 2012) will provide a complete programme to enable you to start working in this way yourself.

This book is written mainly for professionals working with children, either pre-school or when the child has reached school, from support staff to midwives and health visitors, to teachers, social workers, therapists, psychologists, psychiatrists and other medical staff. Foster parents will also find this book useful, although the parent-based style of the other Not Just Talking book 'Helping Your Baby Communicate-from Day One' (Boyce, 2009) may be more suitable.

CONCLUSION

This book is about how non-verbal communication skills develop, from the moment of birth, and how failure to develop these skills contributes to many current social difficulties.

The aim is to make sure that we don't get too far into the twenty-first century without addressing the lack of these skills. If we do, then generation after generation will get further away from knowing how to promote effective communication in children.

For as long as face-to-face communication remains a key feature of human behaviour we will need good non-verbal ability. The conversational skills we take for granted are central to dealing with conflict: without them, relationships and negotiation become more challenging and verbal or physical violence may become more commonplace. But it is possible to turn things around, to develop the skills that are lacking, even in older children and adults. This book explains how.

'MORE THAN MEETS THE EAR'

NON-VERBAL CONVERSATIONAL SKILLS

2

In the introduction to this book, we saw how important the non-verbal side of communication is. To be clear, this book is not concerned with high-level, subtly nuanced skills used in adult life, for instance the slight tilt of the body that subconsciously indicates interest in the opposite sex. These skills are a very high-level feature of non-verbal communication and only develop when the basic skills dealt with in this book – those required to hold conversations – are well embedded.

This section defines what is meant by a conversation and the elements that constitute it, all of which need to be developed by children – they do not occur automatically.

WHAT IS A CONVERSATION?

This might seem an obvious question, but it is important to recognise how far-reaching the elements of a conversation are. So for the purpose of this book the word 'conversation' means any communicative situation where:

1   There is passing of information (the message) between two or more people. Sometimes this information may appear to be one way but in reality it never is. This is because a conversation only works when there is a sender (speaker), a receiver (listener) and a message.

2   All three elements of the conversation have to be equally valued and function equally well. The listener might appear not to be participating in the conversation, but:

3   The listener always has to give feedback indicating their level of interest or understanding. Often this feedback is given non-verbally. Feedback is given even if there is no spoken response.

4   Without this feedback from the listener you do not have a conversation and therefore the message will not be being transmitted effectively.

Conversations happen one-to-one, in small groups or in large groups, as well as on the phone and when sending emails or texts or any other written method of communication. For the purpose of this book, however, I will focus on the spoken conversation.

As you may well have experienced, conversations in other than the one-to-one situation are much more complicated. One-to-one you only have to concentrate on one other person. As soon as the numbers increase, even with one additional person, the skills needed to participate in the conversation are more subtle and complex.

Another difficult communicative situation, which even some adults don't ever feel totally relaxed about, is talking on the phone. Because you are unable to see the person on the other end of the phone, you pay attention to quite small aural clues to understand which words to focus on. These clues indicate how to interpret what is being said so you are able to make an appropriate response.

In the last part of the twentieth century, British Telecom (BT) found that having spent millions on developing their telecommunications software and hardware, people weren't using the phone enough. So they started the 'It's good to talk' campaign with actor Bob Hoskins communicating two or three central facts about conversations:

- women talk more on the phone

- conversations are useful for getting things done

- men have shorter conversations, but should do it more because it's fun!

BT also produced a brochure outlining in a colourful 1990s way the process of holding a conversation and giving many tips on how to get conversations to go well for you. BT continues to support communication-centred programmes and in 2011 is the joint sponsor of the 'Hello' campaign for the year of speech, language and communication (Hello, 2011).

Since the end of the last century, the surge in the number of mobile phones has led to more communication through texting than through speaking on the phone. In the section on what affects our performance in conversations below there is more about why talking on the phone is so difficult.

But for a child it is commonly in larger groups – such as school assembly – when she needs to pick up on signals from more than one person, that her skills become severely challenged. Unless she has developed all the necessary skills, her understanding of what she should do or say will be undermined and her communication level may revert to that of a much younger child.

Even in adult life, such as giving a talk to an audience of a large group of people, we are very dependent on getting feedback, even if it is only a nod of understanding or a ripple of laughter. Many speakers become very uncomfortable when there is apathy or lethargy in an audience (the infamous 'graveyard' slot after lunch, for instance), because it is much more difficult to talk in a situation where there are not active listeners – people who physically demonstrate their interest in what is being said. Speakers will seek out these 'active listeners' in an audience and hope that they are distributed throughout the group, spreading the focus.

Most people are unaware of how dependent we are on the listener to give relevant information. In the Not Just Talking training I include a workshop where people are split into pairs with one being the listener and the other the speaker. Often the speakers think this is the easier role, but within a few minutes it becomes clear that, without feedback from the listener (they are sitting back to back) they become unsure and concerned about how the conversation is progressing. The speaker doesn't know whether the listener has heard, understood or completed the task being communicated. Under these circumstances the speaker becomes disoriented and often just stops talking.

There are many other stressful situations where as adults our communicative ability deteriorates to a much lower level – just like the children. However, being older we have developed more skills and experience, so the drop is not quite as steep and has less impact than it does in a child with fewer skills.

Is teaching a conversation?

Based on this Not Just Talking approach to conversations, all teaching is a conversation – unless you subscribe to the teaching theory of a child being an empty vessel that just needs filling. The approach to teaching in the 1960s, sometimes referred to as 'soft-centred' or 'touchy feely', had one benefit as far as communication is concerned – there was a great deal of interaction between teachers and pupils, and pupils were encouraged to think and speak for themselves.

Nowadays, with the pressures of the National Curriculum, teachers are encouraged to get the children to reach targets and this is sometimes done in a formulaic or 'parrot-like' fashion – although I am fully aware that not all teachers work in this way.

Nevertheless, on occasions I have been told by teachers that conversations are what happen in the playground not the classroom! Unless teachers know that every child in their class has understood what they have been told, then they cannot be surprised if the child appears to decide to do something different. Initially primary school children won't have sufficient skills or confidence to feed this information back clearly, so teachers should make a point of checking that children know what has been said to them and what is expected.

CONVERSATIONAL SKILLS

These are made up of a collection of many different elements – some of which you may not think relate to conversations. As we have already seen, the necessary skills cover:

1   understanding and use of body language and facial expressions

2   interpretation – relating to situational understanding

3   speaker and listener roles

4   reasoning and prediction

5   prosodic skills.

This section will go through each of these skill areas and explain their function within a conversation.

WHAT EXACTLY IS BODY LANGUAGE?

When referring to body language, people tend to think of facial expressions and gestures. But body language is much more comprehensive than this and includes:

1   Facial expressions – this includes those expressions which overtly communicate the emotions such as happiness, confusion, worry, and so on; and the more nuanced expressions for attentiveness or disinterest, as well as more complex messages such as sarcasm and innuendo.

2   Looking at faces also tells us the difference between men and women. At a very basic level, men and women usually have different hairstyles. Also men have facial hair and, if they shave, their skin can be less smooth than women's. In situations of confusion it is possible to combine information from the hairstyle with whether or not the person shaves their face or has a beard, as well as the tone of voice, to establish with some clarity whether you are talking to a man or a woman.

3   Body language – with our bodies we can communicate straightforward emotions. Think of how different your body is when cold to when it is laughing or jumping up and down with excitement or standing rigidly with fear. Both facial expressions and body language also include those subconscious elements that as adults we use to communicate such things as whether we are from the same background as others – see Robyn Skynner's explanation of this in Families and How to Survive Them (Skynner & Cleese, 1993) – or, through our pupillary reflexes, whether or not we like someone. As stated elsewhere, this book is not concerned with the development of these more advanced skills, but readers should be aware of their importance communicatively. These subtle and complex skills are an automatic consequence of developing the baseline non-verbal skills discussed here.

4   Gestures – these are 'informal' automatic hand movements which are made alongside the spoken word, such as automatically opening your hands out wide to communicate the size of the fish that got away!

5   Gestures can also have a more definite meaning than this, such as when waving goodbye or beckoning someone towards you. These are gestures which are used in a more structured way and mean the same thing to all the people who share the same language and culture as you. They can vary between different languages or cultures. This is where confusion can arise. HSBC advertisements have understood the fundamental importance of non-verbal communication because they see it as central to good business practice, for instance showing the soles of your feet in Thailand or a flat, palm outward shove of the hand in Greece, which are offensive to the Thais and the Greeks but which would not be problematic in the UK or USA – see HSBC (2002).

6   There are also other high-level involuntary gestures that we all use, such as touching the throat in embarrassment or touching our head to show regret. These gestures will only develop following good understanding of situations and the acquisition of empathy.

7   Body position – think how much the position of your body communicates non-verbally, for instance if you are lying down or getting up or standing on your toes.

8   Body posture – whether you are relaxed or tense, head bowed or raised, leaning towards or away from someone or something, arms folded or not, and so on.

9   Tension – this is dealt with separately because it is very important in terms of recognising the feeling or level of emotion in a person. The simplest way to explain this is to think of the act of pointing at something or someone. Here are two examples to illustrate this – the point is that even if we can't hear what is being said, the degree of tension in the body will communicate the different emotion:

- A teacher wants the children to look at the rabbit that one child has brought into the class. So she says in a gentle but assertive manner 'Look at the rabbit'. At the same time she points her arm and index finger in the direction of the rabbit. This arm will be relaxed, slightly bent and definitely not stiff.

- A teacher wants to point out to children the mess that they have left despite being told earlier to tidy it up. This time she will say 'Look at that mess!' but the voice will be different to the first example – there will be a brisk and slightly angry tone now. But there will also be a visible change in the pointing arm as it indicates the mess. This arm is now straight, stiff and tense.

There are many advertising agencies who understand the power of this non-verbal communication and there is a wonderful Yellow Pages advert from around 2000. It starred James Nesbitt and is a story about him being asked by his sister to get his niece's hair cut. He wants to save money so he does it himself. When his sister returns he pretends that a hairdresser has made a mess of the hair and then phones a hairdresser asking them to put it right. When he takes the daughter to the hairdresser, the sister waits outside in the car but can see through the window. His body language looks as though he is remonstrating with the hairdresser, but the words he is speaking are a completely different message about how he knows that she didn't make the mistake with the haircut, but could she please put it right? You can see this for yourself on You Tube (see Yell Group, 2003, or just search James Nesbitt and Yellow Pages).

10 Proximity/personal boundaries – it is from learning about how close to stand when talking to different people that we start to establish our own personal boundary. Different people and different situations require different boundaries. So our boundary with a stranger is likely to be larger than with a partner or friend. We have to learn this through many situations where our parents or others have told us where and where not to stand as well as through observation of others. Sometimes parents and schools do not see it as a problem when a 10-year-old still wishes to cling to adults.

Much earlier than this, a child needs to learn who they are able to stand very close to and also where this is possible – it is not so appropriate at school with a teacher, but at home with her parents it is fine. Also as adults we need to understand the signals that will tell us about the formality, informality, familiarity or intimacy of situations.

11 Body direction – this might seem too simplistic, but I have come across children who had not developed a sense of body direction. We need to know that if a body is moving away from us the back will usually be towards us, and if the body is coming toward us we can see the person's face. This applies to knowing which way a queue is going and is particularly important for group understanding – especially in classes, where all the children might not be appearing to go in the same direction, but the child needs to be alert to the general direction of most of them.

12 Hand movements are crucially important as well, because they give us a great deal of information. Think of the following differences:

- putting a coat on a hook and taking it off

- lifting something up or putting it down

- taking a jumper off or putting it on

- doing up shoelaces or undoing them

- closing the lid of the saucepan or looking inside to see if the potatoes are done.

These are just a few examples – we don't even think about it when we are looking, but the message is being received and understood at a subconscious level. For instance, if you see your partner putting on their coat you know that they are nearly ready to go out with you, and the conversation will be about what you are going to be doing. However, if you don't know the difference in the visual clues between putting on a coat or taking it off, you will not know what the conversation is likely to be about. Children who haven't learned this need to be taught it – I have had to teach 14-year-olds this skill.

13 Touch – how we touch each other and what touch means within a communication is another important aspect of body language for the child to learn.

14 Relationships – it is most important that we know something about the relationship of the person we are speaking to, with regard to both ourselves and to other people in the situation. Are they related, or friends, or strangers? There are clues from which we can make this judgement, and this is how it is taught in the Not Just Talking intervention:

- family look similar but are generally different ages

- friends look different but are generally the same age

- strangers are people we have never seen before or have not been introduced to.

15 Clothes and equipment – these communicate a great deal because it is not only what people are wearing but how they are wearing clothes that gives off many non-verbal

signals even before you have spoken to them. Here are a few examples from hundreds that a child needs to learn about:

- uniforms communicate what the person is going to be doing: nurses, doctors, dentists, pilots, shop assistants, postman, funeral workers, etc

- whether we are wearing smart or casual clothes, school, work or home clothes, etc. This last set of clothes is very important in order for children to recognise whether the situation is likely to be at home or in school

- equipment tells us if it is a plumber or an electrician

- warm clothes in the winter or summer clothes

- wedding clothes and other formal occasions

- swimwear

- wet or dry clothes

- sports clothes – these communicate what sport you are going to play – horseriding clothes being different from football kit or tennis clothes, for instance.

Think of your attitude if a man comes towards you in the dark wearing a policeman's outfit. Would your reaction be the same if a man came towards you in the dark, wearing a hood and jeans and you couldn't see his face? This is just an example of how much is communicated through our clothes.

All these clues are important but not definitive; without them you will be confused, but if you depend too much on them you may end up with the wrong conclusion – never judge a book by its cover! What these skills do give you over time is the ability to know where and when not to use them.

Now think about the way we wear clothes and what that communicates:

- Smart clothes but worn in a shabby manner. For example, if a girl goes to a school in a smart uniform, but arrives with her shirt and tie hanging out or her trousers looking like she has slept in them, would her teachers think that she is ready to work hard?

- Smart clothes worn in a manner that communicates that you are not on your way to work, for example, but on your way home. This is because when we leave for work we tend to look very smart, but at the end of the day a man might have taken off his jacket, loosened his tie or rolled up his shirt sleeves.

- Any clothes where the sleeves are pulled up or rolled down communicates something – either that the person is hot or cold or that they don't want to get their sleeves wet. The precise message that is being given depends on other (situational) clues.

16 Age – this is also a very important part of interpretation to get right. A child who talks to her peers and her teachers in exactly the same manner will not be popular, particularly by the time she enters secondary school.

In my experience of children who have entered the Not Just Talking intervention programme, virtually all of them were unable to tell the approximate age of the person they were looking at. This was because they had not learned to read clues such as hair colour or complexion, and to understand their significance in relation to age.

We need to know the age of the person to give them appropriate information – getting both the content and the style correct.

As you will see from all these different elements relating to body language, there is a great deal to learn before you can make sense of the multiple indicators in a specific situation. First we need to learn how to recognise these signals in others and then we will be able to make use of them all appropriately – most of the time. And only by learning the most common interpretations can we learn to deal with the exceptions.

INTERPRETATIONAL SKILLS

The next element of a conversation is how we interpret what is happening. On the basis of this we can predict what will happen next and be able to have some idea about what the other person or people want to hear or say. So correctly assessing what is actually going on is a vital first step.

Situational understanding

First, we need to make sense of the people in the situation, and all the information discussed in the section on body language above will assist in this task. Next, we must be able to interpret the scene or the circumstances – where is it? At home, work or school? Is it a hospital room or is it outdoors? If so, whereabouts? A surprising number of children are incapable of this element of interpretation.

Finally, to make good sense of the situation, we must weigh the first two pieces of information against our previous experience of similar events and locations. This is called the 'experiential' part of interpretation. Because we accumulate more experiences of situations every day of our life, these skills continue to improve as we get older.

In order to make the best interpretation of what you see, you must combine the information gleaned from these three sources. It is vital that equal weight is placed on each aspect because, if one dominates, the interpretation may be skewed. To help illustrate this, here is an example from one of the children I have worked with:

Think of a situation where there is a man dressed in a very smart suit. It is a lovely day and he has a broad smile on his face. He is in his late twenties. Taking account of his clothes and his level of happiness, most people would think that he has just been offered a job or that he may be at a wedding. He is definitely not just going to the sweet shop. We know this because our experience of similar situations helps us narrow down the number of options of what he might be doing. We are taking account of all the visual clues and all of our experiences of similar situations.

However, a child with an interpretational problem looking at the man might think that he is smiling because he likes ice cream. This is a very basic example of the child projecting her personal experience too much on the scene: because she likes ice cream, she applies it to this situation. She hasn't taken into account the fact that he is wearing a very smart suit and there is no sign of him eating or having eaten an ice cream.

The result is that she will talk about ice cream and everyone else will talk to him about his new job or the wedding. As adults, if the clues don't definitively tell us that, for example, this man is going to a wedding or has a new job, then we would ask a question to help clarify the circumstances. Children with non-verbal communication difficulties do not know that this is how we get to the right interpretation, leaving them with only a mistaken or partial understanding.

At a more complex level, it is very easy to get people's intentions wrong if you have only some of the information available. The Guardian newspaper used this idea of making the wrong interpretation without the full story – called 'Point of View' – to advertise the paper during the 1990s. The advertisement showed a skinhead running along a street. From one perspective it looked as though he was running from a car; from another it looked as though he was going to steal a briefcase from a man; but once you had the full picture, it became apparent that he was running to save the man's life by pushing him out of the way of a falling crate of bricks.

In situations where marriages break up and need support from an objective third party, the couple might seek the advice of a counsellor. Counselling is focused on putting back the information that we interpret subconsciously and stating it explicitly. This ensures that the parties are all talking about the same thing.

How we interpret the situation tells us what to say, feel, think and do. So children who have not acquired this ability may be left with a profound sense of alienation.

Connecting information

Once we have made good interpretations of situations, then we need to start cross-referencing experience from one situation to another. This is called generalisation and will help us make good sense of what we are talking about in new and different circumstances. Children who can't do this are unable to generalise communication or learning – it can be seen in autistic spectrum disorders. However, when children's interpretation skills improve they are able to generalise in all areas of their lives, even those on the autistic spectrum.

Rules

An outcome of being able to interpret situations is that it helps us build up rules for how to behave. So when we arrive in a garden centre and it is closed but there are chairs laid out facing one way, we sit on the chairs and keep quiet and listen to the talk on gardening we've come to hear. If we hadn't got this many-chairs-in-lines-facing-a-speaker 'rule', or hadn't interpreted the clues well, we might have thought that we were there to buy plants.

Children who behave in unusual ways may be doing so because they are applying a different rule to everyone else. For example, they take off their shoes and socks because they usually come to use the swimming pool at this venue, but today they are going to see a puppet show so need to apply different rules.

SPEAKER/LISTENER ROLES

The speaker and listener role is very different to the speaking and listening skills which apply to the understanding of speech. These roles in effect are the 'job' that the speaker and listener have to do within the conversation to ensure that the conversation is maintained for as long as is necessary. Speaking and listening skills are about how to understand and use language for communication purposes. We have to have both sets of skills, but for the purposes of this book the focus is on the roles.

A conversation will die without each party possessing good skills in both these areas of development. The children treated by the Not Just Talking method of intervention tend to have problems with both these roles, but the listener role is the more important to develop. Without it the child will not learn what a good speaker does.

What a listener does

So what does a listener need to do? We all probably know that we need to look at the person we are listening to. But what does that actually mean and how do we really know someone is listening? Here is a brief explanation as there is more on this in Section 5.

1   The listener needs to look at the person – not their eyes, just their face, so that they can see the whole body in their peripheral vision. This allows them to perceive the facial expressions and the body language to help make best sense of what the speaker is saying.

2   They also need to be relatively still. A person who fidgets or who moves about is much harder to talk to.

3   The listener needs to demonstrate interest in what is being said.

4   The listening element is a bit easier as an adult because our experience of listening (and speaking) will have taught us what works and what doesn't.

5   The speaker will only know that you are listening if you talk about what they are talking about.

6   Finally, the listener has to give feedback – this can be either verbal or non-verbal, but they need to let the speaker know whether or not they are following what is being said, need clarification, need more or different information, and so on.

7   This feedback includes asking for help if the listener becomes confused. The ability to seek help, to ask for clarification, is most important because in every conversation we are learning about how to understand the next conversation a bit better. If the listener lacks the ability or confidence to ask for help then their skills will not grow in the required manner.

So a listener has to be active, and this is done almost entirely at a subconscious level as most of it is conveyed through small changes in facial expression which, as we will see next, have to be picked up by the speaker.

What a speaker does

The speaker's job is to ensure the message is understood by the listener. To do this they need to look at the listener so they can pick up the feedback that tells them whether the listener:

- has understood, ie, the vocabulary is right

- needs more information

- has had sufficient information

- needs different information

- needs clarification

- is confused.

It is the speaker's role to make sure the message is adjusted to make it clear so that the listener will understand. The speaker will only know how much information is required by watching the feedback given by the listener. This is more complex in a group setting as some listeners will require less information than others. A higher-level skill is knowing how to balance this within a group conversation; it is one of the reasons why groups are so difficult for children with poor non-verbal skills.

Looking versus eye contact and gaze

The difference between looking and eye contact is that eye contact is something that is done to 'get to know someone better', to signal a particular level of interest in another person, and to reciprocate that interest. Generally, this skill is acquired in the teenage years so that you get to know someone of the opposite sex. It is a development made when many other conversational skills are in place.

In day-to-day conversations 'eye contact' is not generally necessary – people know how uncomfortable this level of interest can be under the wrong circumstances. We often need to look at people when holding a conversation and as adults we generally look then look away at regular intervals. However, when people look away for too long while telling you something, this is also very noticeable and uncomfortable for the listener. Under these circumstances you may be bombarded with information that you don't require because the speaker is not tuned into your feedback, telling them you have sufficient information on that subject. Or it may signal that they are more interested in talking for its own sake than imparting a message to you.

Gaze is very different and serves another purpose in communication. It is simply the act of moving your eyes towards an object, event or person. We can direct the person's attention to look at the object, action or person that we are telling them about by using our gaze. We also, of course, can do this in other ways such as pointing at the subject of conversation – 'Look at his red sports car'.

For the purposes of this book, we are interested in just one of these aspects of eye contact – that the child looks at the person/people they are engaged with in conversation.

INFORMATION-GIVING SKILLS

In a conversation we need the ability to know how to give the right information required in the conversation, taking into account all the circumstances. Getting the quantity of information, the level of detail, relevance, style, etc all correct depends on participating effectively in the conversation, especially with regard to:

1   being able to use our interpretation skills well, as outlined above, to pick up the non-verbal signals telling us whether our listener is interested, is following our drift or needs clarification – (more on this below)

2   our understanding of shared knowledge.

This ability to process the signals that indicate what information is required in a situation is vital as it will mean that on entry to school a child will be able to judge how to help her teacher know what she is talking about.

Sharing information

This is different from shared knowledge in that sharing information means that you don't just give information to your listener but ask them for their opinion or add information to the conversation. This enhances the quality of the exchange, makes the listener feel they are part of the conversation and increases their interest.

If the speaker allows the listener to give their opinion, or if they have experienced or seen the same kind of situation, then the listener is participating and will want the conversation to continue. Children who lack this skill find making friends very difficult.

What happens when a person can't give information?

We've probably all noticed people who, when interviewed on TV or the radio and asked a question, even an open question, give a one-word reply. This makes the interviewer's (ie, speaker's) job very hard as they will have to keep repeating the question or asking different questions in the hope that the interviewee (listener) will be prompted to give more information in return.

Some people do this on purpose but others do it because they don't know what information is required. When you find yourself in a similar situation as the questioner, just be aware that a child might not be able to give information.

Initiating communication

The first step is to know what it is you want to say or what the listener wants to hear. This depends on the level of your interpretational skills, your understanding of the shared knowledge you have with your conversational partner and your prediction of how they might react. Without all these skills, the next part of initiating communication will be beyond your skill level. Message initiation also includes knowing 'how' and 'when' to say what you have to say.

The first thing that we need to learn is 'how' to initiate. We have a thought about what we want to communicate to someone. Then we find that person and engage them communicatively. At a basic level this may be just saying 'Hello, how are you?' or approaching that person with a facial expression that communicates that you have something to say. If they are on the ball they will engage automatically with you and it is then easy to begin to convey the information that you have for them.

Many children develop the first skill of going up to people but then do not have the ability to initiate a conversation. As a result, these children may be labelled 'attention-seeking'. They may 'hang around', interrupt inappropriately or become physically disruptive because they haven't acquired the skill of initiating a conversation in an appropriate and timely manner.

Another aspect of being able to initiate is knowing how to request information. This is often a response to the type of information given by a speaker – a request for something further to make the message clearer. Or requesting information may be eliciting specific details that you know the speaker has, for instance, asking a ticket collector at the station when the next train is due.

Knowing when you need to ask for help or need some information that will enable you to make a decision is a key conversational skill. Knowing how much information to give someone depends particularly on your interpretation and prediction skills. These tell you what the listener probably knows about the subject and whether or not they are interested, engaged or confused, and so on. If you are looking at the listener you will know how they are responding to you. Then you will be able to end the conversation or take your part in it appropriately – perhaps becoming the listener in turn.

Maintaining and ending a topic

Remember, knowing how to initiate is the first step, but maintaining and ending the conversation are quite separate skills. The end of the topic is signalled through grammatical elements as well as prosodic elements such as intonation pattern beginning to lower. But knowing when to end the topic is also, as with most of these skills, picked up from the feedback given by the listener(s).

When they have understood or when they have sufficient information, it is time to end. It then might be the listener's turn to take up the speaking role or your job as the speaker to initiate another topic. The situation and the other person's feedback will inform this decision. During a conversation, the decision-making process is constant – what to say, how to say it, when or whether to say it.

Part of the role of the speaker is to make sure that what is being said is appropriate to the listener(s). See below on 'styles' of communication for more about this.

Turn taking

Turn taking is a much more complex skill than I was led to believe when training to be a speech and language therapist. In those days we were told to play board games to help children know how to wait their turn.

Think about the clues that tell you when it is your turn to talk. These are nearly all non-verbal signals:

1   There is a pause.

2   The speaker looks at you.

3   You recognise from the intonation pattern that the speaker is about to finish what they are saying and that there will be a pause where you can take your turn.

4   The speaker points at you.

5   You are introduced to the group by the speaker and they turn to you.

6   The speaker makes a facial expression that says 'It's your turn to talk'.

7   The speaker puts their hands on their hips and looks at you as if tired of waiting for you to speak.

8   There is a questioning intonation pattern – 'Hungry?'.

9   The speaker asks a direct question – 'Where are you going?'

10 Another verbal clue would come from the predicted order of words and their grammatical function, the vocabulary, syntax or grammar. For example, if you heard someone saying 'Would you …' you are likely to know that the person is asking a question. You might even predict what follows: '… like to go swimming?' This would prepare you to give an answer. However, if you didn't pick this up because your understanding of grammatical structures was not sufficiently developed, then you

would have to wait until the end of the utterance and have less time to get your answer ready. Prediction, as you can see, is not only a huge skill with regard to non-verbal communication but is vital for our language skills as well.

You will see just from these few examples the complexity of recognising and piecing together these non-verbal and verbal clues. You have to be able to use all these to ensure that you can take your turn appropriately. This is hard enough in a one-to-one situation, but in a group you have to keep watching and listening carefully to everyone so you recognise all these 'turn to talk' clues – a much more demanding task. If you miss the particular cues because you weren't looking at the right person, ie, the speaker, then you might miss your turn.

If you don't know how to do this as an adult, holding any kind of conversation becomes difficult and this will affect your ability to make friends, hold down a job and, as a result, will impact on your confidence levels and self-esteem. To succeed as adults children need to develop confidence in these skills, something which many today find more challenging.

Negotiation

Being able to negotiate with others for things that you may want or need or to get yourself out of trouble is a skill that we develop through our everyday experiences of situations and observing conversations. Without good conversational skills, negotiation is not possible. Only when a speaker has succeeded in mastering these skills, will she learn through her experience of conversations how others negotiate. She will then apply this to similar situations and so, through years of experience of conversations, she will know how to negotiate at times of joy and trouble.

This is a very high-level accomplishment and is only developed when all the other conversational skills referred to in this book are in place. Even then, sometimes as adults we find negotiating really difficult. Think of hostage negotiation situations. The people who are brought in to negotiate in those complex situations are highly trained experts.

Styles

During conversations with different people in different situations your style of speaking will change. Throughout the day this will encompass many conversations and style changes. The specific approach you adopt will depend on:

- how well you know the person – stranger or friend

- how intimate you are with someone – partner or family

- whether they are a peer, for example, at work or in sport

- whether they have a higher status, for example, a police officer or a judge or royalty

- whether the situation demands a change, for example, a court or church

- whether you are worried or anxious, for example, in hospital or on a plane

- whether your job demands it, for example, customer services, nurse, MP.

These are just a few examples of things that can influence your use of different styles and in reality we might change our style as many as 10–20 times a day. However, if you have only one or two styles available to you because that is all you saw or learned as a child, then this will limit your ability to participate in conversations effectively as an adult. It is very limiting for children too, as without a range of styles, they will talk to everyone in the same manner.

When you are aware of this and start to listen out for it in children, such as talking to the head teacher in the same style as they talk to their classmates, it can sound quite odd. It may be acceptable or amusing to hear in Key Stage (KS) 1, but when a child gets beyond this early age and enters KS2 or 3, it begins to sound less appropriate. It is also much harder to deal with – by this time the child will only improve with intervention. They might also upset people without understanding why.

REASONING SKILLS

Drawing conclusions

Another skill fundamental to conversational performance is the ability to draw conclusions from the information you see. At a basic level this is just noticing that in a group situation people are – for instance – sitting waiting for a train rather than a bus.

At more complex levels there might be a group of people sitting in smart clothes in a waiting area, looking a bit anxious, maybe one of them looking at the clock. Because the setting looks like an office, you are likely to draw the conclusion that this group could be waiting for an interview. Because of their anxious faces there are certain topics you might not broach with them. This leads directly into the next reasoning skill of being able to predict.

Here's an example of the way different interpretations can impact on everyday life:

Think of a train journey where there are five coaches but only one is designated a 'quiet' coach. It is mid-morning and the train is not busy.

If your interpretation of 'quiet' was sitting reading or meditating then you might choose this carriage.

However, would you choose this carriage if what you wanted to do was to talk to a companion or talk on your mobile? Presumably one of the other four coaches which don't have this designation would be more appropriate. But what would be the thoughts of those who had chosen it for the correct meaning of 'quiet'? Would they be happy with the noise?

As long as you draw the correct conclusion 80-90 per cent of the time and, in situations that are complex or unclear, you can ask for help to make better sense of what you are seeing, then your non-verbal communication skills will support you.

Children who have not developed the ability to infer within conversations should not be expected to be able to do so when they have learned to read. They might learn the technique of reading, but will be unable to 'read with meaning' because of an inability to draw a conclusion.

Prediction

When communicating with others the ability to predict is vital on many levels. We need to know:

1   what they want to hear, based on shared knowledge

2   how they may react to the information that you give.

Based on what you interpret from the person's body language, the situation and how you relate it to similar experiences, you then need to adjust what you expect their thoughts, words, actions and feelings to be. It is not necessary to predict with unerring accuracy, but you need to have a good idea what they may do or feel so that you can adjust your communication appropriately for the situation.

Choose appropriate options

When we have interpreted the situation well and managed to draw an accurate conclusion about what is happening, we then have to trawl through (at a subconscious level) our experiences of similar situations and narrow down the several options for what might be the best behaviour and communication.

Only if we have a selection of options can we go on to evaluate which is best for the particular situation. If we are lucky – or skilled enough – we choose the correct one. For children this skill is not usually in their repertoire and they might have only one option, which may work in only one in 10 situations.

Hidden meanings

One of the subtlest parts of verbal language is 'hidden' meaning or metaphor. This leads to a rich and fascinating language that can throw up opportunities for poets to wax lyrical and comics and satirists to have a field day. ('Field day' is itself a 'hidden' meaning, a metaphor using the military term for a day when troops have manoeuvres or exercises, generally used to mean a time of exciting activity or success.)

However, it can be a nightmare for those unable to get beyond the literal meaning of words. Children may also struggle to make sense of hidden meanings because comprehension of the message is only complete if you understand the message behind the words.

If someone says in the right circumstances 'You've got a chip on your shoulder', it needs to be interpreted in the correct manner, ie, someone is quarrelsome or has a grievance. However, if only the words are listened to and the situational context is not applied, the person might look at their shoulder to find a 'chip'.

So the context or other non-verbal information in the situation tells us whether or not this message has a hidden meaning. Imagine you are out on a long walk and the person behind you sees your socks down. 'Pull your socks up,' they say: the meaning under these circumstances would be literally to do that. However, if the person was way in front and you were lagging behind, then it would be likely to mean 'do better', 'get a move on'.

These hidden meanings become much more layered or obscure when sarcasm or innuendo is added. Sarcasm is generally used as a put-down: the face and body communicate different messages. To compound this complexity, the message is hidden behind the words. So telling someone that they are 'such a genius' when the situation is obviously communicating that this person is not a genius, needs the recognition that the words themselves are not actually carrying the message and that, in this case, tone of voice and facial expression play a key role in changing the meaning of the words.

Innuendo again requires us to understand that something else is being requested. 'Wouldn't it be nice if the door was shut?' is a request for the listener to shut the door, or 'You are not made of glass' when someone is blocking the view of the TV, can be deemed to be a less aggressive way of saying 'Get out of the way'.

The common thread to all these hidden meanings is that, in order to understand them, the listener must have good interpretational skills. In secondary schools sarcasm is frequently used as a 'nicer' way of saying something nasty. Whether it has an impact depends entirely on the child's ability to understand these hidden meanings.

In speech and writing this is also known as metaphor – something which stands for something else. Imagine what you would make of phrases like 'time is running out' or 'he's just letting off steam' if you couldn't see beyond the literal meaning of the words.

PROSODY

Prosody means all the supra-linguistic features that help with understanding the message – intonation, stress, rhythm, volume and rate. These are all high-level skills and as such generally do not require support through the Not Just Talking intervention. These skills develop naturally as a by-product of the intervention.

However, in adult life these prosodic elements are most necessary, particularly when listening without the benefit of being able to see the speaker. People with poor sight become very focused on these elements of speaking. These auditory signals communicate a great deal, beyond the use that sighted people make of them, if you can't see the emotional state of the person.

Prosody is also there to help us know which words are the important ones to listen to. Our brains cannot process language at the speed we speak – about 120 words per minute. For years speech and language therapists have worked on the 'information-carrying' words to help children's understanding of language. It is these prosodic elements that are there to direct us to the words that matter most, just like the landing lights for an aircraft. If the aircraft follows the lights it will land safely, so if the listener takes the prosodic pointers to the important words they are more likely to understand the message.

Learning a new language is a way of understanding the importance of these features. If you have learned French or German, for example, you may have been asked to listen to the radio in French or German in an effort to improve your understanding. You are unlikely to benefit quickly from this because understanding of the prosodic elements of that language is not, in my experience, taught as part of language courses. Without this skill you will be trying to listen to and understand all the words. Your brain will become overloaded and you will not have the ability to make good sense of what you hear. Only much later, or if you are able to immerse yourself in the new language, will you get over this hurdle.

Children with non-verbal communication difficulties have this problem but in their mother tongue. They listen to all the words and as a result can't make sense all the time of what we say to them.

Intonation

The intonation pattern helps to not only communicate emotion – a flat intonation demonstrates a lack of interest whereas a lively intonation communicates enthusiasm – but also gives weight to parts of the sentence to help the listener know which words to pay attention to and which are not so significant. It even indicates when the speaker is about to finish talking. This helps the listener know when it is their turn to speak.

Stress

Stress is very important and varies from language to language. This is why even though English speakers may learn all the grammar and vocabulary they need in order to speak French (or any other language), unless they learn the stress pattern and other prosodic features of French, they will always sound as though they are talking good French but with an English (or American) accent.

Stress gives emphasis to a part of the word that is important and again points the listener towards the important things to listen to and away from the words that are not so significant. So it is an important skill for listening to the radio or communicating on the phone.

Volume and rate

Getting the volume and rate correct depends on your non-verbal interpretation of the situation. You need to understand when to increase volume, such as if you are in a crowd or surrounded by other loud noise which makes it difficult for others to hear you. To be quiet you need to recognise that you are in a library or that there is a baby trying to sleep, for example. You may well know of children who tend to shout a lot. This could be a failure to pick up the signals telling them how loud or quiet they need to be and/or the only style of communication modelled to them while growing up.

How do we know when to talk fast or slowly? Again, through non-verbal interpretation – if you see that the person is in a hurry to leave then you may need to speak quickly in order to deliver your message, or if the person doesn't speak your language, you may need to talk a bit more slowly to help them understand.

Children I have worked with tend to err on the side of talking too loud and/or too fast. Once their non-verbal understanding improves this tendency reduces to an appropriate volume and rate for the situation and people.

Rhythm

In English we have what is generally referred to as a stressed-timed rhythm. This is developed through the wealth of nursery rhymes available – although they are not used so often nowadays by parents with their children. In other English-speaking countries where English might not always have been the mother tongue, different patterns of rhythm are used. For instance, South African English has a 'rat-tat-tat' or syllable-timed rhythm. However, as speakers use the other prosodic features of speech in the same way as UK English speakers, this doesn't sound too odd.

But if a child does not acquire rhythm – and this can happen in severe cases of autism or Asperger's syndrome – then they will develop a syllable-timed rhythm, which without a good intonation pattern tends to produce a monotonous tone, sounding more like a Dalek.

So rhythm is just another element of prosody that helps our understanding of the language. All these elements combine together to support our non-verbal communication skills and ensure that we can deliver and receive messages in all situations.

WHAT AFFECTS OUR CONVERSATIONAL PERFORMANCE?

Even when we have a good set of conversational skills, there are still times when our performance is impaired. Because communication is such a complex skill and takes so much of our brain power to function effectively, it is one of the first things to deteriorate under the following conditions.

Tiredness

Most people recognise that when they have had a long day at work, they will need a period of 'wind down' time before engaging effectively in conversations. This is a phenomenon seen in children when they return from school. Most parents realise that they need to sit and 'chill out' in front of the TV or with a book and a snack before they are fit to communicate effectively. This is because concentrating hard and communicating is tiring. The same applies when we are ill. If the body is not functioning well and it reduces our energy then our communication is affected too.

Speechmark

Confidence

In order to communicate effectively you need confidence and, at the same time, being able to communicate effectively gives you confidence. The better your interpretation becomes the more confident you will be about your communication, and thus you will kick-start the process of developing confidence which in turn improves conversational ability.

Good communication will also help build self-esteem. Children entering the Not Just Talking intervention programme almost always have low self-esteem, but most improve significantly, purely as a result of improving their non-verbal conversational skills.

Stress and pressure

If you were to imagine a really stressful day at work, perhaps some or all of these things could have happened:

1   A major piece of work that you were involved in was lost on the office computer system and as a result you had to start again from scratch.

2   Your boss told you that at the end of the week she was going to have to let someone go and decide between you and a colleague.

3   You had a phone call saying your mother was seriously ill in hospital.

Then you go home and it is pouring with rain, get to the door and find you have left your house keys at work. I suspect that you might be feeling slightly stressed by now. Under these circumstances your ability to communicate effectively will inevitably deteriorate.

Children who sufferer from poor interpretation and understanding feel this stressed – often throughout the day – and consequently their already poor communication deteriorates further. Under these circumstances they are likely to resort to behaviour (as adults would do if they were very stressed) as a means of dealing with the confusing situation. They might lash out, withdraw, have a tantrum – whatever works for them in the moment.

Pressure occurs in any situation where you are doing things far beyond your capacity to cope. This could be pressure of too much work or too many things going on at home. For children this includes academic pressure. Wherever the pressure comes from it will impact on their non-verbal communication and cause it to deteriorate.

Why is talking on the phone more difficult?

Any situation where you cannot see the person speaking is harder to understand because you are not getting the total amount of feedback available. Listening to a radio is slightly easier than talking on a phone because as a listener that is all you need to do. You do not have to think of what you might reply when it is your turn to talk.

When BT found that men didn't like talking on the phone as much as women they used the Bob Hoskins advertisement to try to turn this round. However, the reason that men are not so keen on talking on the phone is because of the high-level non-verbal skills needed to do this. Baron-Cohen (2003) says that the communicative differences between men and women do not apply to all men and women. I would agree: there are many men who, given the right opportunities, develop good non-verbal understanding and as a result are more empathetic.

But Baron-Cohen points out that men haven't got the same connections in their brains to facilitate ease of development of these high-level skills – some manage it, but not all develop sufficient skills to be comfortable talking without visual feedback.

My prediction is that forms of communication with visual feedback such as Skype and FaceTime will, in the next few years, become the dominant method of communicating with phones, principally because being able to see the person provides more clues to help make sense of what they are saying.

When communicating on a phone without the benefit of visual feedback, the listener has to work much harder. Not only does the listener have to pick up the auditory signals given by stress, rhythm and intonation to help them understand what the speaker is saying, they must also give vocal or verbal feedback to help the speaker know that they are still listening. The speaker can't see the listener and is getting no feedback from their face or body about their level of interest. So the listener has to communicate this at regular intervals throughout the conversation – much more often than in face-to-face conversations, for instance, 'mmm' or 'Yes, I understand' or 'Oh!'. The speaker has to listen hard for these vocal signals and be able to interpret through the tone of voice or intonation pattern whether or not the listener is keeping up or is interested. It is still the speaker's job to make sure the message gets through in a manner suited to the listener. This is why so many cold calls go wrong. The person calling has a script to get through; they often talk far too fast and they are not making automatic adjustments for the needs of their listener.

CONCLUSION

In this section I have covered what is meant by a conversation and all the aspects that are necessary to make the conversation go well. A conversation will die if one side of the communication partnership is not playing their part well.

The most important feature is the interpretational skills. Without them you will not know what to say, when to say it or whether to say what you were going to say. They will help your life prospects and make life experiences happier. But these skills are of little use unless you know how to be a good listener and speaker. We looked at the difference between listening skills and the listener role and between eye contact and looking for non-verbal information.

The relevance of sharing information was discussed and the difference between sharing information and shared knowledge highlighted. This then led to the skills of being able to start, maintain and end a topic appropriately. Styles of communication aid the process of communicating effectively in all situations and therefore play an important role in keeping the conversation going.

Reasoning skills, such as being able to draw a conclusion from what you see, not only help in conversation but also allow us to read with meaning. Prediction skills are so important communicatively because they allow you to have some idea of what is going to happen as a result of what you say – in terms of how the listener may respond.

We saw the complexity of hidden meanings, which depend on our ability to understand the message behind the words. This is achieved through our non-verbal interpretation of the situation. Then the importance of the prosodic features of communication were discussed, highlighting how vital these non-verbal communication skills are in relation to listening when you are unable to see the speaker.

Finally, we looked at the impact of stress and pressure on the communication situation and how there is a circular link between confidence and communication.

Next, we will see what has changed in society to stop these skills from developing in the way they should.

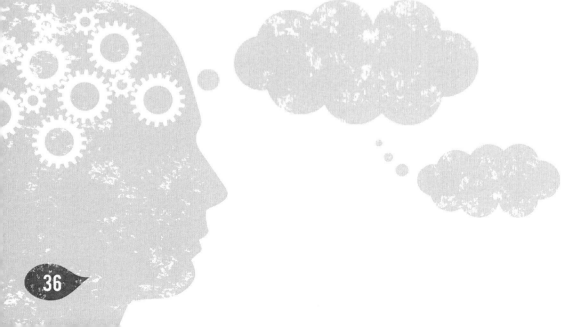

■ 'A CHANGE OF FOCUS' ■

THE CAUSES OF NON-VERBAL COMMUNICATION PROBLEMS 3

As explained in the introduction to this book, the major influences affecting children's ability to develop sufficient non-verbal communication skills emerged in the 1980s. This section will look at the effect of some of these changes.

■ WHAT HAS BEEN GOING WRONG?

The buggy

Before the buggy, babies were pushed around in either a pram or, as they grew, in a pushchair. The benefit of these modes of transport for babies was that they meant that the baby faced the person who was pushing them.

The introduction of the buggy (or stroller) made life easier for parents. I remember the thrill of thinking that getting it in and out of buses or cars would make our lives much easier. Also we all thought that, if a baby looked out at the world, he would become fascinated with what he saw – and more intelligent as a result!

But because he now had his back to his mother, he was not observing her engaged in everyday conversations. At the time no one knew how important observing people in the process of communicating was to the development of non-verbal communication skills. No one wrote about this aspect; the focus was on how to develop verbal language skills and when the child would say his first word. So parents were not able to make an informed choice about such things as buggies; nor were they given advice on how to compensate for the effects of this key change.

It's probably the buggy more than anything else that has reduced the amount of time babies spend watching people hold conversations. Sitting in a pram a baby can see the person pushing him and, most likely, whoever she might be talking to. In a forward-facing buggy, the baby will at best see only one side of the conversation.

Once you are aware of this, you will be surprised how often you notice people pushing babies in a buggy and chatting away to the child while unable to see his face. Babies learn most of their communication skills – both verbal and non-verbal – through watching people who are demonstrating good conversation technique. Talking to a baby when you cannot see his face models to him that you don't need to look at people when you are talking to them.

Think of what people do when they stop to talk to the adult pushing the buggy.

What people might do	Consequence of this action
Bend down and say 'hello' to the baby	Includes the baby in the communication. But the fact that the adult has to bend down so that their face is closer to the baby is indicative of the problems associated with buggies compared with prams – the child is too low down
Stay in front of the buggy and talk to the buggy pusher so that the baby can see one side of the conversation	If the baby can only see one side of the conversation then he will not pick up the subtle non-verbal messages associated with the passing of verbal messages between two people. Also the baby will have to look up a long way to see the face of the adult in front of him
Might include the baby by asking him for feedback such as, 'Do you agree?'	The adult knows that it is important to make the baby feel part of the conversation but this doesn't help all aspects of communication development if the baby can only see one person
Stand at the back of the buggy and talk to the buggy pusher	The baby can't see either side of the conversation and completely misses out on an opportunity to acquire new skills or reinforce rules and skills he has already observed. The baby may become confused because he is unable to pick out who is talking and has no supporting clues to help him understand the verbal language

A baby who is looking away from his parent will need to learn what to focus on, what to look at and what to let go in order to be able to make sense of what he sees. For example he will need to know that a dog is identified by its tail wagging, panting, its size and its bark. If he is not able to identify these defining characteristics he might think that because it walks on four legs it is a dog, or because it has fur it is a dog. So when he sees a cat these features could apply and his understanding would be that this is another dog.

Apply this to more complex situations and you will see how easy it would be to look at the wrong indicators or characteristics. At this young age, the baby is acquiring and honing his perception, but only if he has developed the basic skill of knowing which aspects of the object, person or situation define what they are.

If a child is facing out toward the world in a buggy before his non-verbal interpretational skills have started to develop, he will be looking at everything and will be unable to distinguish what is helpful to him from the profusion of sights, sounds and clues in front of him. Not a lot will make sense to him.

On many occasions I have witnessed the face of a young baby crumple in confusion when is he no longer able to understand what he can see ahead of him. He is confused by what is being said by the person pushing his buggy as they might be having a conversation either on a mobile phone or to other people walking beside them. Young babies particularly need to be looking at their parents to give them a feeling of security and recognition of who they are with and where they are, and to help direct their attention.

I observed a particular incident when walking round a big shopping centre. It was a Saturday and a young couple were out with four friends pushing their baby of less than three months in a forward-facing buggy. This baby's face suddenly deteriorated into panic. The reasons for this were:

- He could vaguely hear the familiar voices of his parents, but he couldn't see his parents at all.

- There were many other voices – including the four other adults talking to his parents – as well as the noise from all the other people in the shopping centre, so it was virtually impossible in this melee of sound for him to keep focusing on the voices he recognised.

- There were hundreds of people milling round in front of him – it was a very busy Saturday morning before Christmas.

- At his age he would be unlikely to have all the skills necessary to make sense of the situation – he would need to be functioning at least a two-year-old level to have a chance of processing all this complex information.

Parents should not be surprised when their child becomes distressed. Instead of just placating him and moving back to pushing from behind, understand why he has become distressed and take him out of the buggy, if there is not an option to turn the buggy round and push that way. Parents often think that children should get back in the buggy. This might not be the best way, especially if the reason for the child using challenging behaviour is his state of confusion.

I have also witnessed many parents remonstrating with their babies and toddlers or cajoling or placating them by telling them they are soon going home or to a shop the child likes. This is unlikely to work if the child has been brought up using buggies and having family meals while watching the TV. His skills of prediction and time sequencing won't be sufficiently developed to understand what will happen in a sufficient range of situations without a great deal of adult support.

Mobile phones

Difficulties posed by mobile phone use when a child is not looking at the person on the phone are fairly straightforward. The reasons why he might not be looking are either because he is in a buggy looking away from the person pushing it or because he hasn't developed the skill of looking at people when he hears speech.

Babies in buggies who hear the adult talking will not have developed sufficient skills to know that the speech may be intended for another person who is not even present! Because babies haven't yet developed the ability to understand complicated grammatical structures and, when very young, depend on the intonation pattern more for comprehension purposes, hearing adults using complex sentences is just confusing.

Moreover, because he is alienated by this confusion, he becomes less interested in what people are saying and this significantly reduces his inbuilt drive to find out what someone is talking about. The lack of curiosity will make him less and less able to communicate effectively.

SOCIETAL CHANGES

There have been profound changes to society since the last part of the twentieth century and little research to evaluate the effect on the development of basic skills in children. But when looked at from the perspective of the development of non-verbal communication, it is easy to see why these changes have had such a significant and detrimental impact.

How did the family meal table help?

Babies and toddlers need as many opportunities as possible to observe people holding conversations – on different topics and using different styles. One of the best opportunities for this is the family meal table. Until the 1980s most families ate together around the table, and this was the perfect arena for the development of non-verbal conversational skills in babies and toddlers.

However, since then family life has changed, so that many families do not as a rule eat together at the meal table. If they do eat at a table, there may well be a TV nearby for people to watch while eating. We are no longer modelling to our babies and toddlers that you need to look at people when communicating.

Conversational skills

Observation at the family meal table also helps the child pick up the non-verbal messages telling him when it's his turn to talk or what others feel about what's being communicated, their level of interest, their need for more information or if they have heard enough.

Additionally, he will learn about different styles of communication, how close people who know one another are when communicating, how people touch one another and other key features of conversation. Because a baby is sitting watching many exchanges, he will also see people communicating in different ways – happily, sadly, enthusiastically, secretively, angrily, and so on.

As a result he will learn that he needs to talk to people in different ways according to the person, the situation and what they are talking about. Babies who see only one style of communication tend to communicate in a limited fashion. Therefore every day he should have the opportunity to watch and listen to all these things in a variety of styles of conversation.

Parents should be made aware of sitting at table participating in a family meal as a key opportunity for children to acquire many essential non-verbal skills. They might then go back to at least providing one meal a day at the table.

Screens

Screens have started to be a 'childminding' service for parents while they busy themselves with the daily routine. Babies are put in front of the TV watching DVDs that parents are told will promote the intelligence of their baby. This is of dubious value since the sheer act of putting a baby in front of a TV for more than a few minutes denies the child the opportunity to learn about daily life just through being with his parents while they do the washing, talk to a neighbour or fix the bath taps. Children need to hear the language associated with daily activities repeatedly so that they can use it appropriately in situations away from home. And observing or participating in everyday routines also increases their exposure to non-verbal communication.

For many years, people have been concerned about a link between violence on TV (and other screens) and poor behaviour in children. The main area of concern has to do with children watching programmes that contain violence, bad behaviour or pornography. If this happens before they have developed sufficient non-verbal skills to be able to process what they see, they won't be able to tell reality from fantasy. Therefore they cannot be blamed if they copy what they have seen. This imitation of behaviour in a 'parrot-like' manner is done without understanding the consequences. Of course, this also applies to any behaviour witnessed at home – such as violence between parents or siblings, inappropriate sexual relations, and so on.

Throughout the period from birth until teenage years, children are accumulating increasingly sophisticated skills that will help them make best sense of the more bewildering situations they will encounter during the transition from teenage to adult life. Parents should not assume that children have the skills to interpret these complex situations before they are in their late teens. In the past the censor rating of films and the nine o'clock watershed served this function and parents took heed of them. Because parental and social attitudes have changed and children are now able to view things that are beyond their interpretational skill level, they do not understand that what they are seeing is not reality.

Children who see screen-based items of a violent or sexual nature may well use this behaviour in another situation for these reasons:

- their interpretation of the situation is limited so they may apply behaviours that are inappropriate for the situation

- their prediction skills are poor and therefore they do not understand the consequences of their behaviour.

Play

Children play outdoors less nowadays owing to concerns for their safety. This has had a knock-on effect regarding communication development. Because conversational skills need a great deal of practice in different situations with peers, the lack of opportunity to play outside with friends is a serious impediment. It needs to take place before the child reaches school so that he will be able to cope in the playground.

Travel

The fact that we now depend heavily on our cars and don't walk as much as previous generations of parents also limits the number of conversations a baby can watch. The car seat has been developed with the focus on safety. Rear-facing car seats in the front are a good choice because the baby is able to look at the face of the driver, but before long he grows too big to stay in the rear-facing seat. Also they cannot be used in a car that has airbags that can't be switched off.

Once the child is in the back seat, he is no longer able to see the face of the driver or others in the front seat and as a result they are modelling to the child that it is not necessary to look at people when talking to them. The use of the car also reduces the number of occasions babies have to observe two or more people holding a conversation. Walking or taking the bus offers many more opportunities for a baby to watch conversations.

Extended family

In the past family mobility was less common – people tended to work and live in the place where they grew up. This meant that grandparents and aunts and uncles were on hand to help a couple with childrearing. This is particularly relevant with the first-born child and his non-verbal communication development.

When parenting responsibilities were shared between generations there was closer family interaction in general. All of this meant that the routines and techniques that help reinforce non-verbal skills were constantly used and passed on. Nursery rhymes and games played a big part in parenting.

Nowadays things are very different and many new-born babies live far away from their grandparents or other relatives. It then becomes a lottery as to who the parents have contact with and whether or not those people are able to model the best way of promoting non-verbal skills. As generations go on, those new parents who haven't developed sufficient non-verbal skills as children are less likely to promote them in their own children.

Shopping

When I was a little girl, I remember going shopping to Sainsbury's with my mother, but not as we know it today. In the 1960s the shop that we went to was in two sections –

one side was interconnected with the other but each side of the shop had different counters for bacon, cheese or dry goods – biscuits, and so on. At each counter you would queue and watch the conversations going on between the assistants and the customers. The customers would talk to one another in the queue too. Because the number of shoppers was smaller, we would meet the same people most weeks; they probably came to the shop more than once a week or on the same day each week as transport was not so available.

Today, not only do we walk round supermarkets with trolleys (which do have the baby facing the right way!), not really having to talk to anyone, but also shopping is increasingly done online. Communication in these types of shopping situations is very restricted – paying at the till or telling the driver where to put the shopping bags when the delivery van turns up at the door. Again, opportunities for babies and toddlers to watch conversations are severely diminished.

BENEFICIAL CHANGES

Experiential opportunities

Potentially, now there are many more experiences for children to have than before the 1980s. So theoretically, non-verbal communication skills based on the experiential aspect of the child's life should be really good. But this is not the case because children no longer learn to look effectively for information in a way that will help them in processing this information for use in another situation.

Childcare

As far as learning non-verbal communication skills is concerned it doesn't matter who teaches them to the child. Parents who go out to work should not worry as long as the childminder understands the importance of developing these skills. Childminders, foster parents and adoptive parents are all well placed to promote non-verbal communication so that the child becomes an effective communicator.

Special care

A newborn baby being in special care does not in itself prevent the development of early communication skills. However, if the parents or midwives are focused on the development of bonding it is easy for the baby to miss out on the development of interest in faces – an essential precursor to developing all other conversational skills, and to bonding itself.

Nursery provision

Many nurseries do well with regard to giving visual clues to children, but sometimes there is an over reliance on children choosing before they fully understand what a 'real'

choice is – see Section 12 on intervention. However, nurseries are an excellent breeding ground for conversational skills and, as long as staff are fully aware of the need for children to develop basic skills such as prediction, turn taking, information-giving and sharing, then this should set them on the road to doing well at school.

After-school clubs of all types

Again, these clubs offer really good opportunities to expand conversational skills. However, it all depends on the child having developed sufficient ability before he goes to the club. If his skills are poor, his behavioural difficulties are likely to result in the club refusing to take him as he may be disruptive to the smooth running of the club.

CURRENT PROFESSIONAL ADVICE TO PARENTS AND CARERS

The advice from midwives to bond with baby, although well intentioned, can lead to frustration and depression in parents as it is not easy to bond with babies who are not developing good communication skills. These skills are the foundation for the development of bonding, thought and language and as such should be the first focus for midwives and health visitors.

Most advice given to parents is based on developing language skills. Parents are told that as long as they talk to their babies, all will be well. But hopefully by now you will realise that this is not the whole story. Talking to the baby is important, but more important is that the baby has many opportunities, each day, to observe two or more competent conversationalists talking. Only then will the child develop the skills necessary to be a good communicator.

This 'talking to' your baby or toddler produces situations such as the following, witnessed in the queue for a till:

> A grandmother had come to the till with her grandson who was about nine months old in a forward-facing buggy. She had accumulated all the items she had selected on top of the buggy and was putting them on the conveyer belt. Behind the conveyer belt was a pot of flowers to tempt people to make a last-minute purchase. The baby couldn't see those because she had directed the buggy at an angle away from the till.

> She was making a particular point of telling him exactly what she was doing (in line with the current advice). However, the boy was not only looking away from her because the buggy was not facing her but he was completely distracted by something going on a till or two away. His grandmother had no idea that all the words she said were completely wasted because she couldn't see his face. He had no idea that she was talking to him. It was a real shame, because what she was saying would have been extremely helpful not only to his conversational development but also his language development. This is what she said:

> 'Shall we get these lovely flowers for mummy?'

> 'Mummy will love them, won't she?'

CONCLUSION

In this section I have covered the main factors that, as a result of changes in the past 30 years, have reduced the number of opportunities children have to develop non-verbal communication skills. By school entry a child should have developed all his verbal language skills but, more importantly, he should have developed to a high level with regard to non-verbal skills.

Without this development, he will not be able to go on to acquire other skills over the course of his life. Remember, this is the only communication skill that has to develop every day of your life in order that you become better and better at communicating with ease in most daily situations.

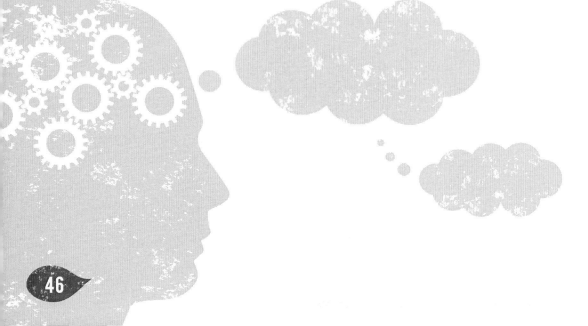

■ 'COMMUNICATION CONTROLS THE WORLD' ■

BABY DEVELOPMENT 4

This section will show how the development of non-verbal conversational skills pre-dates the development of language, and how without them children cannot make full use of their verbal language. Non-verbal communication skills not only underpin the acquisition of language but are also a precursor to the development of bonding and thinking skills.

In the past it seems to have been assumed that babies are born with the ability to communicate non-verbally, ie, to read facial expressions and body language, to interpret emotions and contextual clues. In reality babies are born with a propensity to develop non-verbal skills, but these will only mature if they are promoted by those in contact with the infant and until the child enters school and beyond.

There has been much research over the past 10–20 years into what babies can do in the first weeks of life. Babies are fascinated by faces, but research has shown that this instinct to seek out faces may only last for the first 24 hours of life. Research has also shown that a newborn baby is so 'programmed' to look for faces that, despite his vision not being fully developed, he is able to look at them and copy movements such as poking out tongues and moving eyebrows! However, no one appears to have asked the question, 'Why do they do that?' When faced with the problem of children who could talk but not communicate, I began to investigate these earliest instinctive attempts at communication and gradually the significance of this 24-hour period became apparent.

In due course many of the other things that babies were seen to do made excellent sense in terms of the development of non-verbal communication skills. This section will show how these apparently unrelated skills are the bedrock of communication development and how, when they fail to develop, children go on to be able to talk but are unlikely to communicate effectively, causing them to struggle in many everyday situations.

■ THE NEW BORN BABY

Babies are born with natural instincts and reflexes to do certain things. Here are some of the reflexes that a baby should have in the first few hours and days of birth:

- Rooting – when the baby's cheek is stroked, he will turn towards the side being stroked.

- Sucking – put a teat in the baby's mouth and the sucking action starts automatically.

- The palmar reflex – the start of being able to grasp items.

- The Moro/startle reflex – when the baby is suddenly not held, his arms and legs will automatically open outwards.

- The plantar/Babinski reflex – when the underside of the baby's foot and toes are stroked, they will spread open.

There are also other events during this period, many of which are directly associated with the acquisition of communicative ability.

The very first act for a baby is to breathe. This is followed by the first cry, which is a reaction to air rushing into his lungs. This first breath is encouraged by the delivery team by sucking out any mucous in the baby's airway and, if this doesn't start the first intake of breath, as a last resort they might slap his feet or bottom to jolt the baby into breathing and crying. This makes sure that the lungs fill with air. As the air is pushed out of the lungs by the baby, ready for the next breath, the vocal cords start to vibrate, hence the cry or scream. Both these events are vital for speech later in the baby's life. You need air going in and coming out of your lungs to talk and the vocal cords give you your voice. The baby will have to use his vocal cords and lungs a great deal to ensure that he develops the fine control necessary for speaking.

The rooting and sucking reflexes are precursors to eating skills. Because these muscles are the same muscles used in speech, these reflexes are also precursors to the spoken word. The rooting reflex gets the baby in the right position to suck, which will exercise the organs of articulation (lips, tongue, soft palate, etc) for increased control. A high level of control will be needed later to make the fine movements necessary for complex speech sounds in sequences and at speed.

Even a small word such as 'back' requires a very high level of control and 'programming' by the brain. The vocal cords need to vibrate at the same time that the lips come together for the /b/. Then the vocal cords stay vibrating but the mouth opens in a particular way for the /a/, and finally the vocal cords have to stop and the back of the tongue rises to meet the soft palate for the /k/ sound. This is how much control of his organs of articulation the baby will need to develop in order to speak just this one word, let alone a message of 30 seconds. Just starting this at the right moment requires intricate processing and timing by the brain.

So these newborn actions are important for later speech skills, controlling the breath and vocal cords so the child will be able to change the shape and position of different parts of his vocal tract to make a variety of speech sounds. These sounds will later be combined to form words when language is present.

WHY ARE FACES SO IMPORTANT?

The first 24 hours

The most interesting and essential action that a baby makes at the moment of birth (after breathing, of course) is that he is driven to look for faces. This drive only lasts for

24 hours and so we might ask ourselves: 'Why is this such a relatively short period?' A possible explanation is as follows:

Imagine a baby being born in the middle of nowhere with only a mother and father present. They are young and it is their first baby. Without extended family to demonstrate differently, they may not engage with the baby in the way that is necessary.

However, if the baby's first instinct is to look at faces, then the parents will be prompted to look back at the baby. This response to the look of the baby kick-starts the process of developing communication.

Once the parents take control they will continue to look at the baby's face, communicating with the baby through facial expressions and vocal noises that will help calm the baby – and may also get him excited about what is going to happen (I will say more about the importance of the skill of anticipation later in this section).

Ramsey-Rennels and Langois (2007) report that it is agreed by most researchers that newborn babies have an interest in faces. But there is disagreement as to what drives this interest and which facial expressions a baby can interpret (Farroni et al, 2007). However, what is important is not which expressions a baby knows but the simple fact that he will develop such a strong interest in faces that he has an opportunity to learn what different expressions mean both to others and for him.

In my experience, babies can copy facial movements in the first hour of life. For example, if someone sticks their tongue out while looking at the baby's face, the baby will start to do the same in response! At this stage a baby's vision is not sufficiently developed to focus on smaller features, such as mouths or eyes. But this desire to look at faces is so strong that the baby is able to mimic what the adult does. (The faces are usually quite close as the loving parents wonder at this new life.)

I have often recommended to parents that they encourage their newborn to do this by poking their tongues out: this very easily generates a response. It might seem socially odd, but in terms of developing interest in faces it works a treat! The baby enjoys it and looks at other people to see if they will do it too.

A baby's natural instinct to search for faces fades after 24 hours unless it is stimulated. So the more parents can encourage their newborn to look at faces in those first few hours after his birth, the better. Nowadays many babies miss out on this critical first stage that is the vital grounding of non-verbal skill development. This is happening largely as a result of higher standards of neonatal care, which mean that a premature baby often goes into special care as soon as he is born. Also babies born by Caesarean section with a general anaesthetic may be sleepy for the first day or two – so might his parents be! All this doesn't matter as long as the parents focus on this skill as soon as they can when the baby is out of special care. It doesn't matter who kick-starts this process – parent, relation, carer, sibling – the important thing is that it happens and that it is passed on to others, for instance, if the midwife manages to develop the interest in her face while the mother sleeps, then shows the mother what progress has been made and talks about the benefit. If the person who is the main carer of the baby doesn't appreciate the importance then the baby's interest will die away. (Parents should also remember to keep promoting facial interest once the baby is happy to look at them.)

Perhaps surprisingly, this interest in faces can be encouraged at any age (I have managed it with 14-year-old autistic students), but it is necessary to work much harder and longer to establish the child's interest in faces.

What this process of looking at faces does is to make a connection with the parent. We all find it hard to resist responding to a baby when he looks straight at us. The action of looking at the baby encourages him to look back and thus, almost without having to think about it, we have the start of interaction. Once this has happened it is then the adult's responsibility to continue looking and responding, thereby passing on to the baby subconsciously a habit that will enable them to acquire all the non-verbal skills the baby will need in order to communicate effectively.

The most important thing a parent can do for their baby's communication development is to make sure that he learns that faces are exceptionally interesting. Between the day the baby is born and the day he enters school, he will have to look at hundreds and thousands of faces to learn the subtleties and differences between the communication of the same emotions in different people. Moreover, he also needs to have watched many examples of two competent conversationalists – adult or child – talking to one another. This is the reason why at this stage of development the baby should be strongly encouraged to develop his instinctive interest in faces.

HOW TO PROMOTE OTHER NON-VERBAL SKILLS

There are many things that go to make up the non-verbal skills that babies need and, as long as parents can make the connection between these and the emergence of spoken language later in the child's life, they will be keen to make sure their baby is competent in all of them.

Introducing signing

Before a baby can understand words, he has to rely on making sense of facial expressions, gestures and tone of voice. But these are sophisticated clues and it takes some time for babies to become really good at interpreting them. Because he does not yet have the skill or experience to interpret them fully, he is not always able to make good sense of what is going on around him. Signing will help bridge this gap between what he sees and what he can understand until he is able to make better sense of the world.

If the baby thinks that being put back in the car after leaving the supermarket means that his parents are taking him to another shop, he may throw a tantrum if he really wants to go home. However, if he has learned the sign for 'home' parents can use this to help him understand that home is where they are going, and this will mean the likelihood of a tantrum is much less.

When a baby of, say, three months cries, it can be hard for parents to work out what he wants. However, if he is understanding some really useful signs, such as 'nappy', 'drink', 'book' and 'snack', then parents can offer him choices and he will indicate which one he wants.

So it is really important to start using signing very early, almost from birth. A baby needs to have many opportunities to see the signs linked with the situation or object and the spoken word so that he will learn what the signs mean. Parents tend to think about introducing signs when the baby is approaching three to six months because in their minds the baby won't be able to use signs until he has got the hand skills to make them. But the sooner he sees the signs, the sooner he will start to make the connections between the sign and nappy changing or bath time, and so forth. Among many other important communication skills (speaker and listener roles, start and finish, etc), the complicated skill of making connections is being practised as well. Learning to understand and use signs before three months – before he talks – also means that his conceptual development and understanding of language will develop much earlier.

The earlier the baby can learn to understand what is going on the better. In Not Just Talking: Helping Your Baby Communicate – From Day One (Boyce, 2009), there are two chapters about the introduction and use of signs. There it is argued that because the baby is not going to use signs beyond the development of spoken language – as speech is a much more effective method of communication than signs – it doesn't matter what signs parents use with their child since the signs will disappear between 12 and 24 months. Only if the child has some other diagnosis that means language and speech will be delayed beyond three or four years will it be important to use an established sign system.

So signs will form a vital link between the time when he is unable to understand spoken language and the time when spoken language begins to make sense to him. Without this understanding parents will find their baby more challenging as there will be limited 'real' understanding of what he wants. At this stage, signs are the key to opening up communication for the family.

Bonding

Today professionals working with parents, both before and after the birth of their child, emphasise the importance of 'bonding' with their babies. Of course, this is a very positive message to give new parents, but bonding is only possible through communication. In the past the baby's non-verbal skills were promoted almost unknowingly by parents and carers, and as a result bonding could be established more readily.

When the baby misses this vital 24-hour period in which he has the urge to look for faces, parents might find that they have a quiet, undemanding baby. But trying to bond without developing non-verbal communication is a bit like asking a baby to run before he can walk: if the baby has missed out on the essential first step towards full communication, he will find bonding more difficult.

EARLY DEVELOPMENT OF NON-VERBAL COMMUNICATION SKILLS

A baby is born with a few reflexes that will set him on the path to develop all that is necessary to be able to walk, talk, eat, learn to draw and write, and so on. However, as with those skills that relate to walking, there are many low-level precursor skills that the baby needs to acquire in order to be able to progress to more complex abilities later in life. A child will not learn to walk if the muscles in his legs don't develop sufficiently and in the correct manner to enable them to support and move in the required manner for walking. Similarly, with communication, parents should recognise and take advantage of opportunities that occur in the first few weeks to develop the baby's fundamental skills such as anticipation, use of his voice, speaker and listener skills, and the rest.

The development of thought

Non-verbal communication development will be the foundation for the development of his thought processes as well. These skills underpin so many areas of development that researchers should start to look at their benefit to the baby. Peter Hobson (2002) in his interesting book, The Cradle of Thought, reports that:

- There is currently no theory that covers the development of autism. Researchers are nearly at a point when the central key to autism will be unlocked, but this has not yet happened.

- If one central cause could be identified it would make the diagnosis easier and it might be possible to do something earlier to rectify the problems of autism.

- Researchers recognise that the roots of autism are in what fails to happen in the interactions between people.

- He also is concerned that autism cannot be diagnosed in the first year of life.

- A new approach is required.

I am confident that research into the development of non-verbal communication skills at this stage of a baby's life would make a valuable contribution to answering the questions he poses.

What the child needs to be able to do

A child needs to maintain the interest in faces that he has at birth. He needs to be able to recognise the difference between a wide range of emotions, including happiness, sadness, boredom and anger. He also needs to understand different degrees of emotion – are people sad or distraught? He must be able to recognise the differences – and the similarities – in the way different people express the same feeling. If he has learned to do all this by the time he meets his first teacher, he will recognise when the teacher is becoming slightly annoyed and will change his behaviour so that she is happy with him.

Think what might happen if a five-year-old spoke to his teacher in the way he speaks to his eight-year-old sister. Imagine what might happen if he doesn't recognise when his teacher is first beginning to feel irritated by his behaviour and only takes notice when she has got to the point of being furious with him. Life will not be easy for him.

If a child is to learn these skills by the time he is four or five years old, as a baby he needs to look at hundreds of different faces making hundreds of different expressions. Babies and toddlers need to see as many adults as possible making exaggerated happy, sad, bored and angry expressions – exaggerated because babies learn to distinguish these feelings only if they are loud and obvious. Parents should remember how easy it is to change what they do with their baby to promote these essential skills – make sure that he is interested in looking at faces.

Without the early development of the basic skills described in this section, the child will fail to develop the more subtle non-verbal conversational skills that will help him develop and make use of spoken language as he grows up. It is the adult's job to give the baby support to know what he needs to look at and what he can ignore.

Interactive skills

Interactive skills are based around the cues and signs that get a conversation going, maintain it for a suitable length of time and end it at the appropriate moment. Of course, we don't all get this right all of the time, but developing these skills makes sure that between 80 per cent and 95 per cent of the time we can hold effective conversations. Before the baby learns to talk, he will develop many skills that will underpin his ability to interact in a conversation.

The importance of feeding

This whole process starts – after the development of interest in faces – with feeding time. When a baby is breast-fed, interaction happens naturally as the baby sucks and pauses to catch his breath. Breast-feeding has long been advocated on the basis of the bonding and nutritional benefits, but we can now add interaction as another highly beneficial outcome.

However, bottle-feeding can also offer the same opportunity, as long as parents are aware of the importance of pauses in feeding to allow opportunities for to-and-fro interaction. It is also important that the baby is fed in a position where the parent is looking at the baby's face at close quarters. A baby feeds in spurts, and during the pauses the parent is able to return the baby's gaze and gradually develop this small communication into something increasingly rich.

At first, there are only smiles or other facial expressions used by the parent and watched by the baby. Then, in time, the baby starts to take part in the process by making sounds or facial expressions in response. Parents should take this as a cue to allow the baby to lead the 'conversation'. By this I mean rather than simply giving information through their facial expressions, words and noises, they begin to copy what the baby has done. For instance, if the baby smacks his lips together, then that is what the parent does, or if the baby makes a longer gurgling sound, then the parent copies the gurgle using the same intonation pattern.

Parents need to help their baby realise that what he 'says' is interesting to them. This is achieved through imitating noises he makes as if replying to him in a conversation. Copying the baby like this is called 'mirroring' and will let him know that his parents value his attempts at communication even though they might not always understand what these early efforts mean. It will also encourage the baby to continue the 'conversation' by offering other communications for his parent to imitate.

Give and take

A key element of this early development is to give the baby the skill of being able to initiate a communication spontaneously. Too often, in my experience, children arrive at school being able only to receive information; they find giving or requesting information very hard. But parents can help develop this crucial life skill from the earliest exchanges with their baby.

Another conversational skill that this interaction starts to develop is that of turn taking – knowing when it is your turn to talk. This is the foundation of the 'give and take' nature of conversations – knowing how to participate without dominating. Parents will know that their baby is starting to take turns when he understands that if he does something and then waits, his parent will copy his sounds and leave a space for him to add another sound.

From simply mirroring the baby's communication, parents move on to the next stage by extending the communication. This is achieved by modelling for the baby how the exchange can develop into more varied or extended ways of giving and receiving messages. At this early stage the changed response may be as basic as replying using a slightly different sound. Here is an example: when the baby gurgles at the parent, the parent can gurgle back but using a different sound or different sequence of sounds or intonation pattern, each time progressing the 'conversation'. This can be done at any time, not just feeding.

These exchanges should be playful, and sometimes the parents will lead, sometimes the baby will lead. This will encourage his ability to initiate communication as well as to respond. Parents will want him to be an independent communicator so they need to stimulate both sides of the communication process.

A baby needs to learn about the 'give and take' of conversations before he learns to talk. He will do this by knowing how to:

- start a conversation

- wait his turn

- respond to others.

These skills are the basis of the role of speaker and listener within a conversation. They develop and become very complex skills as baby grows into a toddler. At this baby stage these skills are laying down the basis of effective communication. Although it is possible to learn them later in life, they are much more difficult to acquire later. Time spent by parents helping their baby at this stage will benefit him in the future.

As the baby grows older, the skills of interacting continue to develop, giving him the ability to take turns appropriately in conversations. He will understand – and take pleasure in – the give and take of successful conversations. He will also become aware of body language and vocal indicators such as stress and intonation to help him know when it is his turn to talk.

PROMOTING INTERPRETATION SKILLS

How parents develop this interest

As already seen in the opening comments of this section, babies are really keen to look for faces. Adults need to make sure not only that can they see faces but that the faces are communicating at a sufficiently exaggerated level so that the baby can't miss them.

In the past few years there has been a movement away from what was seen to be 'baby talk', ie, exaggerated facial expressions and vocalisations. People seemed to think that by talking to a baby in an adult fashion the baby would pick up this way of speaking more quickly. However, we need to work harder than ever to make sure that our babies become good communicators and the best way to do this is to exaggerate expressions and sounds.

A few books provide good sources of photos of babies making faces (for example, Miller, 1998), but photos of real people making exaggerated facial expressions are few and far between. By showing even tiny babies these books and making the faces themselves, parents can help their baby make the connections between facial expressions, not only of different people but also of people of different ages.

Finally, parents should make sure that they get close to their baby so that he can see their face clearly – bend over the cot, get down on the floor with him, lift him on to their knee. When baby gets a bit older and is in a buggy or a bouncy chair, he may be low down on the floor. Encourage parents to step back so that he can see their faces or better still, get down to his level.

Problems caused by the buggy

A baby sitting in a buggy facing out at the world will be bombarded with a mass of visual information. Because he doesn't have the skills to distinguish what has significance, ie, what to look at and what to ignore, he will be very confused. This skill of knowing what to look at helps the baby learn to make good sense of the world.

We've all witnessed a young baby's face crumple into confusion when being pushed in a forward-facing buggy. He can hear the voices of his parents behind them but the mass of visual and auditory signals coming at him is so great that he goes into a state of panic. When prams faced the parents this would have happened less frequently as the baby could focus back on looking at the faces he had already learned about and therefore felt safe and secure.

Similarly, if parents are talking on a mobile while pushing the buggy, the baby has no clue who the parent is talking to. Because the baby cannot see the parent, he is unaware that a phone is involved and is likely to be very confused.

In these situations our expectations of our babies are too great. We expect them to have skills that they do not possess and as a result prevent them from developing the skills they need.

So babies in a forward-facing buggy or in front of a TV, or any other screen for that matter, cannot process the visual information coming at them in huge quantity and at high speed. Babies learn gradually and more easily how to recognise and sift the information by sitting in a pram looking at whoever is pushing it and by watching life in the household, for instance washing up, making the beds, having a bath, eating meals, and so on, where their attention is more directed and focused.

When baby is watching – and especially if people are talking about what they are doing – he will start to absorb non-verbal clues and make associations. Such situations need to be repeated often so that the baby can make connections between them and apply this knowledge appropriately to new experiences.

Screens

Just a brief note about TV screens. The non-verbal clues from body language and situations are too subtle and complex for babies to pick up from the TV. Only in real life situations where parents are exaggerating their facial expressions, body language and vocalisations will babies be able to pick up the distinctions and the similarities between expressions.

Sue Palmer (2006) reports in her book *Toxic Childhood* that research has found that putting a baby in front of a screen too early damages the development of attention. There is also evidence that it will impair their scanning ability for reading. Moreover, time spent in front of the TV is detrimental because it reduces the time available for the baby to be watching and participating in activities with his parents.

Self-awareness

When a baby is born he is unaware that his body is separate from his parent's or anyone else's. He doesn't know where he ends and his mother begins. Gradually in the first year he starts to become aware of others in a meaningful way, rather than the simple stimulus–response relationship that exists at birth, exemplified as: he is hungry–he cries–his parent gives him milk.

Awareness of self is a crucial skill for communication. If we believed that what we had in our brain was the same as another person had, what would be the point of communicating? But if we knew that the other person had different thoughts and feelings then there would be a purpose to it.

Back in 1994, Channel 4 showed a series of programmes called Baby It's You. While most of the essential elements of child development were well understood and established facts, as with much of the research around babies and what they can and can't do, no one thought to relate these developments to communication skills. The programme talked about how the baby doesn't recognise himself in the mirror but first of all recognises his mother or father because he can see them and associate them with the image in the mirror. But, as he can't see himself, he doesn't have this memory of his own image so will look at himself and be fascinated without relating the image in the mirror to himself.

By around nine months the baby will gradually start to develop the ability to recognise himself in photos and in mirrors. This signals the separation of his 'self' from his parents and sets him on the road to wanting to communicate more complex things. This accompanies the psychological development that occurs during this time. Skynner and Cleese (1993) and Hobson (2002) both explain this very clearly in their respective books. Skynner talks about the way a baby in the first year of life has to move away from the protection of his mother. The father's role in the family is to detach the child from the mother and bring him out into the real world through developing communication with his father. Hobson talks about the development of thought and how this comes about through language development. He says that thinking develops through the links that a baby learns to make between his own experiences and those he sees others having. He recognises the importance of the baby learning about the relationship that others have with objects and people. He also sees, among other things, the development of awareness of others as central to language development.

One delightful way parents will know when this skill has been established is when the baby understands that he can make others laugh. This shows that their child is beginning to know that other people think different things to him.

Developing non-verbal understanding

Alongside all of this baby should be developing his understanding of the world in more complex situations. From the start the baby doesn't really know what to look at to make the best sense of what he is seeing, so a parent's job is to facilitate this for him.

Current advice for parents is that as long as they talk sufficiently to their baby, all will be well. This is important, but only if the baby has developed the skills described in this section. Parents should be advised to encourage the child to watch people talking and, as a by-product of this, language will develop in a much more meaningful way. And they should ensure the baby can always see the person who is speaking to them.

The current advice to parents to keep language simple and clear is helpful. Long and complex instructions or commentaries, such as 'I am going to put the dishes here and then I will rinse them before putting them in the dishwasher', may not be understood by any child before the age of about three! Rather, use direct and very straightforward utterances to draw the child's attention to the language he needs to learn, such as 'Let's do the washing up', 'I am rinsing the dishes', 'Now the dishes go in the dishwasher'. These phrases should be repeated until that action is completed. Parents should not confuse the situation by changing the language because it sounds better to them. The whole process should be to model the language that the child is going to be able to use in a manner they can easily access.

Emotional development

The theory of emotional intelligence is well understood – Daniel Goleman (1999) has pioneered this approach since the mid-1990s. But the basics of emotional understanding develop very early and are key non-verbal skills. Currently the focus is on how to rectify a lack of these skills later in life, but it is vital that we enable parents to develop emotional understanding in their child from the earliest possible moment.

How emotional understanding develops

In order to learn to understand his own emotions, a baby first of all needs to recognise in others both the emotion and the cause of that emotion. For instance, his mother smiles because she likes chocolate (happiness); his sister cries because her toy is broken (sadness). A baby will only recognise these emotions if they are communicated in a broad and exaggerated manner.

This is how a baby starts to learn about emotions. (In the next section on toddler development there will be more about the further stages of developing emotional awareness.)

1 The baby sees basic emotions at a very high level – for example, very happy, very worried or very angry.

2 Because the baby is keen to look at people, he will see at the same time what might have caused the emotion, for example, his dad gave his mum a hug which made her smile, or his brother kept on kicking the table and that made his mum cross.

3 People make comments on the cause and the emotion, for example, 'Thank you for hugging me. Hugging makes me feel very happy.'

4 The baby begins to make a connection between the cause, the facial expression and the emotion – as long as he sees this happen a few times and the people talk about the experience in a similar manner.

5 The child then experiences a similar situation. He senses a different feeling developing in his body and this feeling is associated with what he is doing. It reminds him of the emotion he saw his mum feeling. Soon he will start to recognise that this feeling that he always feels in association with that situation is happiness.

6 The more he experiences these feelings – especially with different people demonstrating them to him – the easier he will find it to learn about more complex emotions later.

He will only develop sufficient understanding of what others are feeling if he has frequent opportunities to link facial and spoken expressions to their cause. Showing the baby these emotions in an exaggerated fashion, and as often as possible during the day, from very early on in his life, will help to ensure he is able to associate feelings and their causes.

Remember that seeing these things on the TV will be too complicated for him to pick up readily before he has developed really good communication skills, which won't be until he is at least four or five years old.

HOW A BABY COMMUNICATES

Use of non-verbal communication

It is well documented that babies have different cries for different situations. Five is the most common:

1 I am hungry

2 I am tired

3 I am in pain/discomfort – possibly nappy needs changing

4 I have stomach cramp

5 I have wind.

It is important for parents or carers to be able to distinguish these different messages. However, the cries may become less distinct if the parent anticipates what the baby wants too quickly, such as if the mother rushes into the baby's room and picks him up immediately. Instead she should wait and listen and look. Given the opportunity, the baby's cries will vary. Parents should listen carefully to the cry and try to ascertain what it might be about. Otherwise they lose this opportunity to make sense of what the baby is saying. Parents need to remember that their baby wants different things when he cries and they should listen and not always assume that he is hungry or wants his nappy changed. Of course, if they have been signing to him, he soon will be able to tell them why he is crying and this will reduce the need to cry.

As their baby progresses from newborn, parents should pay attention to what he is looking at. They should talk about what the baby sees in straightforward simple language so that he will have a chance to listen to words associated with what he is looking at, not just what other people have seen.

The beginning of touch

Touching means any touch that happens between two people – it could be hands but also arms and sitting on laps. Nursery rhymes and lap games are a huge part of a baby learning how and when to touch.

It is also one of the first things that parents do with their babies. Touching is a natural part of looking after a baby, through changing his nappy, bathing and rubbing in cream to prevent nappy rash. Through these everyday activities their baby will learn the meaning and pleasure of touch, which will help him immensely later in life.

Babies need to learn what touch means and how to touch others. This continues to develop through to adolescence when it becomes really important to know how to touch people appropriately.

For centuries Indian and African mothers have massaged their babies with oils – this is a practice that is becoming more common in the UK. There are many books about how to massage babies, for instance Baby Massage by Alan Heath and Nicki Bainbridge (2000) and there are courses to help parents do this with their baby. The more touching there is in circumstances like this, the more opportunities there are to learn about how to touch people, as well as many more chances to practise conversational skills as part of the interaction.

Use of signs

Signing is a very important and effective way of developing communication with an infant. If it is started very early (within the first month), first, the parent gets into the habit of using the signs, and second, the baby will learn the signs before he learns how to process the spoken word for the object or action. After he is about six months old the baby will start to use the signs himself to communicate what he wants without having to resort to a screaming fit. In Section 5 I will deal with how temper tantrums are related to poor non-verbal interpretational skill development.

There are certain things a baby must be able to do before he can learn to sign:

1   He must be able to look at faces for more than a few seconds at a time, so that he can learn how to copy the signs being made.

2   He must be able to imitate the actions made with hands or the body. Parents should check if he can wave back at them. Can he copy clapping? Nursery rhymes are another excellent way to find out how well a baby can copy.

3   He must be able to manipulate his hands and fingers well. For example, can he separate two fingers from the other fingers? Or make a pincer motion with his thumb and index finger?

Once the baby has learned to understand the signs, he can be encouraged to make the signs himself – if he hasn't started already! Babies want to communicate with other people and, given an effective way of doing so, they will.

When a baby is screaming in his high chair and parents know that he understands signs such as 'drink' or 'nappy', they can say to him, 'What do you want – drink or nappy?' At the same time, they sign only the words 'drink' and 'nappy'. They should keep things simple by giving him only two options.

He should be encouraged to respond by the parent signing and saying 'drink, yes?' ('yes' and 'no' are important signs for a baby to learn). Then the parents should wait for him to copy them. If he indicates that this is what he wants, perhaps by pointing at the drink or getting excited, they should say his name and sign 'drink'. If he still doesn't sign, they should try taking his hand and making the sign with him, then give him the drink straightaway. This is known as 'proto-declarative pointing'.

If a baby is communicating effectively, the response must be immediate. This teaches him that signing is the efficient way to communicate, and that it can be far more effective than crying. If parents don't respond immediately, he will revert to screaming. But if they do, then the next time it happens he may well sign 'drink' straightaway.

Once he starts using signs, he might very quickly start to combine them, for example 'mummy kiss' or 'drink now'. This ability to combine words will be very helpful when he starts to talk, as he may well suddenly start talking in four- or five-word phrases, with three of the words being signed.

These signs will also be really important in his toddler phase when tantrums start. If he understands and is able to use signs, then when he goes into a tantrum and verbal communication is no longer a possibility, he will be able to follow the signs made to him and may also be able to sign what is wrong.

OTHER WAYS OF PROMOTING COMMUNICATION

Parents should also allow their baby to learn how to communicate non-verbally through nursery rhymes, action games, and the like. They should always respond to the baby's attempts to communicate non-verbally. If these are ignored, like the distinct cries they will disappear and the baby will have to resort to other more physical methods of getting his own way (which are not so good for an easy and happy family life).

What movement does

Once a baby starts to be able to move about, the act of movement itself changes the body for good and there is potential to use his voice and the sounds he makes to a greater extent. There is also a sudden surge in both the communicative opportunities and the language, because he comes into contact with different objects and situations.

At this stage it is still very important for parents to be with him, commenting on what he is doing and extending this commentary to draw his attention to different aspects of what he is seeing or to other items associated with what he sees. The more a baby hears language associated with a situation and actions the more likely he will be to develop an understanding of that situation and what commonly happens.

Promoting language through non-verbal communication skills

Of course, this will have a huge impact on the development of his understanding and use of language. But doing it this way ensures that he will learn to use language with meaning and not just parrot-fashion.

As babies develop non-verbal communication skills, their thought processes and language are developing at the same time. However, non-verbal development underpins these other skills, so, without sufficient non-verbal development, thinking and language will progress less well.

In my experience, even at a later stage beyond the baby period, by concentrating on non-verbal skill development it is possible to improve not only spoken language and thought processes but also memory. This is because non-verbal skills enable a baby to focus on the spoken word in a manner that helps them make good sense, ie, listening to the information-carrying words, not all the words spoken. He is therefore in a learning situation where he is likely to store the knowledge in his language database. If a baby is watching his parents while they are preparing the bath every day and the parent is making sure the baby watches and talks in a style that is clear and unencumbered, the baby will learn a few words to go with the whole process, such as 'bath', 'water', 'towel'. The next thing a parent will notice is that when they say 'We need the towel', the baby will look towards the towel, indicating that he has understood the word. In time, the baby will start to have a go at saying those words too.

In the next section I will be talking much more about the development of grammar, articulation and vocabulary and how these skills improve with the development of more advanced non-verbal skills.

Babbling

A baby is not born knowing how to use his voice. During the period from birth until he learns to talk a baby will have to exercise his vocal cords and all the muscles he will use for speech to ensure that he can start talking between about 12 and 36 months of age. This amazing development is achieved through crying, gurgling, babbling, laughing and cooing from a very early age. All these help him gain fine control of his vocal cords and other organs of articulation, such as lips, tongue and soft palate. Initially this is encouraged by copying any noises he makes with his voice and then extending the range of sounds produced by modelling them to him.

When the baby has developed finer control over his mouth, palate and vocal cords he will start to experiment more with sounds. The first sounds he is likely to have made will be /mmm/ and then when he sits up /ddd/, but gradually /g/ or /k/ will appear as he finds that he can raise the back of his tongue too. Vowels develop naturally around the consonants and then the baby starts to babble, ie, play with strings of /CV/ (consonant/vowels) from about six months, and then moves on to /CVC/ syllables.

These sounds are very different from the early gurgles and coos because they begin to resemble speech. This is because the babble will have the same intonation pattern that is associated with his mother tongue. Babbling will help the baby to develop these patterns so that by the time he is talking he will be very good at using intonation correctly.

THE FAMILY MEAL TABLE

As baby gets older he will start to eat solids and this will change the sitting position and the way his parents interact with him as he feeds. Soon he will be able to sit in a high chair at the table and this will greatly increase his opportunity to observe conversations taking place.

The process of eating is one of the richest parts of a baby's life for developing non-verbal conversational skills. What follows will help people look at the family mealtime in a completely different way and see how beneficial these everyday conversations are. The meal table is central to creating opportunities to talk and anticipate, signal the beginning and end of events, and other conversational skills.

How does the family meal table help?

Sitting at the family meal table while lively conversation is taking place, babies see the smiles and frowns, the looks of surprise that indicate people's feelings. He will notice people leaning forward to show interest, using their hands to emphasise a point, lowering their voice to share a secret – all the varieties of intonation and style that convey meaning and intention.

Babies learn through watching adults and older brothers and sisters who model all these individual styles of conversation. This gives the baby an understanding of how to behave in different situations. One of the most important things to model is that he needs to look at people while communicating.

However, think about how many times a week we sit down together, as a family, without a TV present, and eat a meal. Once a day? Once a week? Never? Only a few decades ago there were three meals a day where children ate with one or both of their parents. In doing so the baby would have an opportunity to watch the whole process of the coming and going of the different elements of the meal.

One of the essential skills for a baby to learn is how to pick up particular clues from people and in his immediate environment which indicate what is about to happen in any given situation. This gives him a start in learning how to behave in different situations. If a family are sitting at the table with a baby or toddler in a high chair and the older members of the family are focused on watching the TV, then conversation takes second place. What is being demonstrated to the baby is that you can eat, talk and watch the TV at the same time without needing to look at the person you are talking to. This is such a high-level conversational skill that only children over the age of about seven are capable of doing it. Until that time, babies and younger children need to look at people while communicating. So, if we all turned the TV off while eating at the table, children would have more chance to be good communicators.

Signalling the beginnings and endings of activities

Babies need to recognise signals that identify the beginning and end of actions and activities. As adults, we do these things quite naturally and unconsciously, but babies and children have to learn them. There are many opportunities to pick up these cues in a structured and well-signalled manner at the meal table.

Prediction helps all children to become confident and happy because they are not anxious about what is going to happen next. Being able to notice the beginnings and ends of activities also helps establish boundaries later on in the child's life.

Think about the process of laying a table. The act of laying the table tells us that a meal is on the way. People understand, when they see that the table has been laid, that the meal will be served up shortly. Sitting the baby at the table in a high chair before parents start laying the table allows him to see the gradual build-up to setting the places on the table before the food arrives. He learns to notice that the meal has not yet started but will be able to predict that it is about to happen. He may also hear his mother or father confirm this by calling out, 'Come and sit down. Lunch is ready.'

The arrival of plates full of food signals the start of the first course. Then, as the food disappears, the baby learns that things are getting close to a finish. Maybe the parents or siblings might say to the children 'finish your food', reinforcing through words and intonation pattern what is going on.

At the end of the first course the empty plates are taken away and, because he sees that there is still a spoon at each person's place, the baby learns that there is more coming. Soon he will learn to predict that it is pudding. It is easy to see that doing this three times a day would be most beneficial.

The number of 'start' and 'end' signals encompassed in just one meal at the table are many and varied. Here is a brief analysis of the stages a baby or toddler will observe two or three times a day at the family meal table.

- Table being laid with the cutlery.

- Layout of the cutlery communicating that the meal has not yet begun.

- Preparing the meal.

- Getting the plates out of the cupboard.

- Calling the family to the table.

- The family sitting in expectation of the food arriving (many non-verbal signals from the family as they do this!)

- Dishing out the food on to the empty plates.

- Placing the full plates in front of the people who are waiting to eat.

- Food being eaten – at first the plate is full and gradually it becomes empty.

- Removing the dirty cutlery and empty plates.

- Cutlery communicating that the meal is half-way through – clean pudding spoons still there.

- Getting pudding bowls out of the cupboard.

- Getting the pudding out of the fridge.

- Dishing out the pudding into the bowls.

- Placing the dishes in front of those waiting to eat.

- Eating the pudding – at first the plate is full and gradually it becomes empty.

- Removing the dirty cutlery and empty plates.

- Lack of cutlery now communicating that the meal is finished.

- Removing all the meal items from the table – salt and pepper, sauces, etc.

- Cleaning the table.

- Washing up the dirty items from the meal.

He will also pick up the verbal communication that goes on between the people. This will include asking questions – 'Do you want chips with your sausages?'; giving information – 'I am going to play with Dean after lunch'; planning conversations such as what might happen at the weekend; sharing information such as what different people think about games they might play or new fads.

This is just a brief analysis of one aspect of non-verbal signals learned at the family meal table. Before about 1980 most children had the opportunity to experience this kind of modelling at least three times a day. If a child is unable to observe these processes and recognise the significance of cues and sequences, he will not be able to predict what might happen next. The ability to predict is a key factor in helping him become confident and happy.

Developing many conversational styles

Because the baby is sitting watching a variety of conversations, he will see people communicating in different ways: happy, sad, enthusiastic, secretive, angry, and so on. In this way he will learn that he needs to talk to people in different ways according to the person, the situation and what they are talking about.

Babies who only see one style of communication (not just at the meal table) tend to communicate in a limited fashion. These are the children who talk to everyone in the same manner – either they shout at everyone or they are very assertive, or shy.

How can feeding help the development of conversation skills?

The transition to spoon feeding should be another step towards a baby's enjoyment of food and eating. As anticipation is such an important communication skill, parents can use spoon or bottle feeding to develop this skill.

With the bottle, parents can bring the teat closer to the baby's mouth in two or three stages. At each point as the teat gets close they can say, 'Here it comes … here it comes … in it goes!'

There is also a great deal of anticipation associated with the use of a spoon to feed a baby as he starts to widen the types of foods that he eats. Parents should first talk to their baby about filling the spoon – 'Look, banana'. As they approach his mouth with the spoon, in stages they should say, 'Here it comes … here it comes … open wide'. Then they can add something like 'yum yum' as the spoon enters his mouth. All messages given to a baby should be accompanied with exaggerated intonation patterns so that the child hears the intonation and associates it with the activity.

Of course, these activities also promote turn-taking skills – the baby needs to wait for the spoon and when the spoon goes in his mouth the 'turn' passes to him. He eats the food and then opens his mouth for the parent's turn to fill the spoon again. Many activities with babies and toddlers can be used to underpin these essential turn-taking skills.

Voice recognition

The baby also learns to recognise the sound of his parent's voice. This started even before he was born because he often heard his mother's voice while in her womb. Then, when born, he hears his mother's voice close to him during feeding, bathing, changing, and so on.

Again, as with all these non-verbal communication skills, it is not vital that the mother or father are the ones demonstrating and encouraging them – anyone interacting with the child can help to reinforce these skills. Being able to recognise and differentiate between voices are important skills, because the baby will start to feel secure if he hears voices that he recognises. Security is really vital throughout our lives and we all communicate much better when we feel secure and safe.

Later, the ability to recognise different voices will help him tell the difference between friendly voices and those of strangers, as well as being useful for communication on the phone.

Speechmark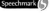

COGNITIVE DEVELOPMENT

Structure and routine

Structure and routine are very important for a baby. They settle him into life by giving key events throughout the day regularly and repeatedly: feeding, playing, nappy changing, bath time, sleeping, and so on. Parents need to signal the beginnings and ends of these activities very clearly so that the baby becomes used to what constitutes bath time or nappy changing. This ability to identify the beginnings and ends of activities is a central communication tool that he will need for the rest of his life. Without it he will find many aspects of communication bewildering.

The Secrets of the Baby Whisperer by Tracy Hogg (2003) is a really good book for parents that outlines all the key ways to structure a new baby's life. Much of what Tracy recommends helps to develop skills for non-verbal communication, even though this is not always explicit. But the suggestions do delineate activities in a helpfully structured manner.

Structured activities can help to draw the baby's attention to the visual clues signalling the beginning and end of activities. To ensure that their baby will learn to recognise for himself the start and finish of activities, parents should signal these points very clearly. Then the baby can learn to identify and pick up the signals that indicate an action is starting or finishing. By this I mean using signs and words to identify the beginning and end of an activity, such as: 'It's time for nappy changing' and 'Nappy changing is finished'. If necessary, parents should point out the visual clues that show the start or finish, such as taking the lid off the jar of food, pulling the plug out of the bath, putting the changing items back in the bag.

Signalling beginnings and endings sits well with talking to the baby about what is happening, what parent and child are doing together. It works best if start and finish phrases are emphasised in a clear sing-song voice.

All this structure and routine forms a platform for the development of many skills, including cognitive skills. Structure and routine will help the baby make sense of a very confusing world.

Imitation

The ability to imitate is important for many reasons, not only ones to do with communication. But if a baby doesn't learn how to do it he will be disadvantaged in all areas of communication development. He won't be able to copy signs, sounds, actions, words and gestures. Without this skill a baby will not develop the ability to do new things.

We have seen that a baby can imitate from birth but gradually starts to choose whether or not to copy what he sees. Babies need to copy facial expressions and hand and body movements as well as things such as sounds, rhythms, intonation patterns and volume.

Anticipation and prediction

The other benefit of structure and routine is that it helps the baby to be happy and confident because it helps to develop his prediction and sequencing skills. Babies are not born with the ability to predict what is going to happen next, but within the first month or two he learns many skills that will ensure that when he is older he will be able to predict from moment to moment and thus avoid the onset of preventable anxiety. Anxiety is a big cause of communication problems, as we all know: when we are anxious, communication becomes increasingly difficult.

Think about applying for a job. There are moments throughout this process when you may become anxious because it is difficult to predict people's responses, from putting in the application and not knowing whether you will be offered an interview, to having the interview and not knowing whether you will get the job.

At a communicative level, we need to be able to predict what people need to know or how they will react in order to give them the right level and amount of information. The ability to predict will develop only if the baby has learned – from experience – to anticipate events.

Parents will know that their baby can anticipate if he stops crying or moves his body in an excited way when they approach. They will only know that he can really predict when he can actually tell them what he is going to do next. So what can be done to help children learn to anticipate and predict?

First, parents should give the baby space to develop this skill. It emerges when parents notice that their baby quietens from crying on hearing the approach of his parent. This tells the parent that he is predicting their arrival in the room and anticipates their face over his cot. Later, he will demonstrate it in other situations too, such as when he anticipates something pleasant is going to happen and moves his body in an excited manner or shrieks with the excitement of anticipation.

Other activities to promote this development in the first few months are based on parents telling their baby everything that they are doing with the baby, for example, putting his trousers on. If the parent:

- tells the baby at the start 'We are going to put on your trousers'

- then repeats while doing this 'We are putting on your trousers'

- when finished, says 'Now you have got your trousers on'

he will hear this pattern of speech many times during a week. Gradually, as he begins to understand the word 'trousers', he might demonstrate that he has predicted what is going to happen through looking at or pointing to or even picking up his trousers.

The use of other indicators, such as 'Here it comes, here it comes', will draw the child's attention to what is going to happen. Combined with a sing-song type of intonation and an increase in the speed of delivery, this helps the child to know that he is going to be given a mouthful of yoghurt or something he really likes. It can also be used with many other activities such as changing his nappy or preparing the bath. Another benefit to his non-verbal skill development is that at this early age his attention is being drawn to intonation patterns and speed as indicators of information that will be useful to his understanding of the situation and what is being said to him.

Of course, another rich source for understanding what is going to happen next is through nursery rhymes and repetitive songs such as 'We're going on a bear hunt'. Games or books are also a good source of opportunities to predict.

This early development of prediction skills will ensure that the baby has a chance of understanding sequences of information and it will stand him in good stead during the next few years of his life, when there is a huge increase in the need to predict in complicated situations. A child who is able to predict will be better equipped to learn because he is less likely to feel anxious or frightened.

Learning to choose

Babies need to learn to understand what a choice is – we have seen that this can be helped by signing and in nursery rhymes and games. When he is a toddler, being able to choose will help all aspects of his communication development.

At this stage parents should just be aware that in the first six months a baby develops the ability to use his index finger to point at objects and people. By the time he is a bit older this skill will help him to ask for things before he can talk.

Once a baby can point at things he will be able to start choosing. Choosing is the ability to weigh up the options and to identify what you want to do. All humans become unhappy and frustrated when choice is taken away. This will help the baby to control his life and ensure that he is happy and content. Choosing is also useful because it will give him the chance to practise both choosing and giving messages – a key conversational skill that only develops with practice.

A baby is not born knowing how to choose. He will need to be given opportunities to learn how to choose. Parents should start early by offering choices of toys, clothes and food and drinks, then move on to choice of games or objects, things to do or places to go.

What change means to a baby

Within a conversation, people, situations and topics can all change many times. A baby needs to learn how to deal with these changes very early in his life. It may also help prevent too many tantrums when he grows into a toddler, because later in his life the ability to cope with change becomes a central factor in whether or not the child can react appropriately.

Coping with change is not as easy as it sounds and a child needs to be able to deal with negative and positive change. Change can cause confusion which leads to stress and anxiety if you can't read the clues that tell you that moving from one thing to another will be all right. He will need to learn how to predict change – this develops from the baby's ability to know when things start and finish. So signalling change in the explicit manner described for beginnings and endings will help the baby to learn to recognise change.

Parents need to know that when change is signalled clearly it should start with something positive. A baby needs to be used to dealing with an enjoyable change first, such as having a treat instead of doing something else less interesting, like taking him to the swings when he thinks he is going to taken shopping.

A baby who finds change hard may cry a great deal, particularly in new situations. A child who can't predict change and deal effectively with it will become over-anxious and may react in unexpected ways.

Early on, parents should use 'Oh dear!' (with an exaggerated intonation pattern) to indicate that a change is going to happen: maybe granny can't come to see him or daddy is going to be late home. They should make a point of linking this to doing something else that is pleasurable: granny can't come, so let's go to the park. They will also need to encourage him to accept disappointment without a positive alternative – he may need to do this often when he gets older.

RESOURCES

Nursery rhymes

People who work with children understand the fundamental importance of nursery rhymes and this is reinforced by much recent research into the development of communication, reading and writing. In the past, nursery rhymes were handed down from generation to generation and mostly people didn't realise how central they were to learning key skills. Nowadays, many children arrive at school having missed out on this part of their development because of the focus on screen-based rather than book- or story-based activities (Palmer, 2006).

Nursery rhymes give babies and toddlers skills for non-verbal communication as well as spoken language. Through the repetition and intonation patterns of nursery rhymes, the child learns a great deal both from listening to and joining in with rhymes and action songs. When the child has heard, on many occasions, people saying 'Round and round the garden' as they trace their finger round his open palm, he will show signs of anticipating the outcome by the excitement in his body before his parent's finger creeps up his arm or they tickle him!

Babies and parents enjoy doing nursery rhymes and lap games – they are fun, help parents bond with their baby and develop his confidence. Parents must ensure that their face is close to baby so should sit him on their lap or in his high chair. From this position he sees clearly not only what their face does but also what their body is doing. They need to find a rhyme or action song their baby really enjoys and then repeat it often. Doing the actions with the rhymes helps the baby pick up the rhyme more easily.

This little piggy ...

The changes to intonation, rhythm and stress patterns inherent within nursery rhymes, such as 'This little piggy went to market, this little piggy stayed at home ...', plus the variations in speed and volume of delivery, are all demonstrated to the baby in a larger-than-life manner by the parent. This is enhanced by the proximity of the parent and the playful manner in which the nursery rhymes are recited, ensuring that the baby picks up these subtle changes more easily and over time will start to use them himself.

Speaker and listener roles

A child can also learn a lot about the roles of speaker and listener, which is covered in full elsewhere in this book. Through the repetition of nursery rhymes he will practise looking at people, sitting still to hear what is being said and listening carefully. They also give many opportunities for a baby to ask for more and to make choices. Finally, of course, the simple act of doing the nursery rhymes on a daily basis with the child encourages him to look at people and get enjoyment and information from doing so.

The importance of 'Ten fat sausages'

This nursery rhyme is brilliant for, among other non-verbal skills, promoting interest in faces and prediction. If parents can interest their baby in this rhyme it will benefit him immensely. This is because he will love the popping sound made by the parent's mouth and little finger!

Here is an explanation of how best to present the rhyme:

Rhyme	Action
Ten fat sausages sizzling in a pan	Hold up ten fingers in front of face
One went (pop)	Make a pop sound with a finger in the mouth – the word 'pop' doesn't need to be said
The other went (bang)	Clap hands or bang on the table – the word 'bang' doesn't need to be said
Eight fat sausages sizzling in a pan	Two fingers are removed. Then repeat the verse, starting with 'Eight/Six/Four/Two fat sausages ...' until ...
There were no fat sausages sizzling in a pan	Make a sad face

This is an excellent intervention tool and I have used it with children of seven or eight and they have loved it and benefited from its facial interest properties.

Books

Parents will find that interesting their baby in books from an early stage is very beneficial, not only in terms of developing an interest in reading but from a communicative perspective as well.

Sharing books really establishes a basic communication skill of passing information from one person to another. The target that a parent should work towards is for the baby to start pointing out things of interest he sees in the book. This will demonstrate that he is developing an understanding of shared knowledge. It shows that he understands the other person hasn't seen what he is pointing out. The act of simply sharing books and games is a starting point for this important communication skill.

The books that really focus the baby's attention on faces and emotions are any that have photographs of people's (not animal's) faces communicating different emotions. The Margaret Miller books already referred to are good, as are other books of baby faces and parents by Roberta Grobel (2002).

The series written by Benedicte Guettier (2004), which have a hole in the middle which the parent can look through at the baby, are an excellent method of drawing his attention to the face. There are many of these and despite being drawings of animals and objects, they work because there is a real face in the middle. Children love these books, especially if the parents are very animated in pretending to be a monkey or a steamroller!

Toys and games

Shared interest

Games offer the same kinds of opportunities to share interest as books, but need to be played in a manner that offers the baby the chance to communicate. Obviously, this becomes easier if the baby is signing. If the baby cannot sign, then parents need to pick up on eye gaze or pointing as a communication that the baby wants an object or picture.

This can be achieved with any game for babies. Posting games are great. If, for instance, the posting game has three objects to post in the holes that correspond to different shapes, then the parent holds on to the object and the baby has to 'ask' for the next one by pointing, signing or vocalising. The parent then gives the object to the baby immediately. Opportunities like this every day really help to hone the skill of requesting (objects or actions) before the baby has developed the ability to do it with spoken language.

Leading activities

Another aspect of non-verbal communication skill development that games offer is for the child to lead activities, for example, in the bath or during play. This is done by encouraging the baby as often as possible to ask for things through pointing or, as soon as he is able, with a facial expression. Parents should always respond positively by giving him what he wants. This will encourage him to try to do it again. Babies need lots of practice.

Communicating 'yes' and 'no'

An important skill that parents need to develop in the child early on in this period is the ability to communicate ways of clearly saying 'yes' and 'no', nodding and shaking his head, for example. This is so helpful in many situations and is particularly useful when choosing. If the child can't nod or shake his head, then pointing or pushing away with his hand would do. In all situations, learning disability or in child development, the basic ability to say 'no' to a situation is a human right. Many children are unable to do it clearly, so are subjected to situations that maybe detrimental to them. By learning to say 'no' he will also learn that he is able to control his environment through communication and doesn't need to resort to behaviour to do so.

Modelling communication

In play, cuddly toys can be used to act as 'go between', for example, giving the toy something like a drink and getting it to hold its paw or hand out in a 'Can I have that' type gesture. Then parents could ask, 'Donald, ask for a drink' and repeat the toy communication if necessary. If this is done on a few occasions the baby will get the idea and start to hold out his hand to request something from his parents or siblings. Modelling other communications with the toy will help the baby start to use the communication himself.

Requesting more

Toys that make a sound are great for offering opportunities to request actions or 'more'. The earlier parents introduce a sign for 'more' the better. The more they use this sign the more the baby will see it associated with the word 'more' and soon the baby will understand the concept. This method enables earlier progress than if the parents had to wait until the baby could say the word 'more'.

The parents should show that the toy has the capability of making a noise – a squeak or an electronic toy is fine. The parent should hold the toy so that the baby can't pick it up and do it for himself. This is not denying him the chance to learn how to make a toy squeak – he will have many opportunities to do that. But it is offering him the chance to develop a communication skill that nowadays may not come around too often.

Then the parents should say, 'Do you want more?' or 'Again?' (with a rising inflection to signal a question). The parent should take even the briefest glance at the toy as a request and play the sound again. This should be repeated for as long as the baby is interested. Theoretically, as soon as he realises that he is in control of the sound it should encourage him to try it many times, as it will be exciting for him to learn that communication controls the world.

Basically, any game or toy can be used in a manner which offers opportunities for the baby to request actions or objects. As long as parents and carers think of games and toys in this way they will find their baby developing good communication skills as a by-product.

UNDERSTANDING LANGUAGE

If parents develop these essential non-verbal communication skills in their children in the ways recommended in this book, they will need to make less effort to promote language development. Language is the natural consequence of developing sufficient non-verbal communication skills.

This has been shown to be the case through the work I have done with a secondary school which specialises in children with severe learning disability, autism and severe behaviour problems. Focusing solely on the non-verbal skills – either in normal development or older children with special needs – children start to talk automatically when a point is reached in their non-verbal communication development.

Conversely, if you promote language skills before the development of sufficient non-verbal ability, you end up with a child who can only use a very few or no words at all, and may also be unable to use the few words that they have with meaning. Without understanding or meaning there is no communication.

If adults talk to babies in elaborate sentences the baby won't be able to make sense of what they are saying and as a result will not make progress. Parents should talk to their babies using exaggerated intonation patterns and short clear phrases. They should only worry about the grammatical structure when the child is putting two or more words together. Even then, they should continue to focus on the development of non-verbal communication skills. So talking to a baby as an adult will not help him develop the ability to communicate with peers and adults. There is much more on this in Not Just Talking: Helping Your Baby Communicate – From Day One (Boyce, 2009).

CONCLUSION

This section has concentrated on the skills that should develop normally from birth until about 12 months and how parents and carers can encourage them. These skills begin developing from the moment the child is born and need to develop to a very high level before baby starts to talk, as they underpin the development of language.

We also looked at some of the things that hamper non-verbal development during this phase of the child's life before he talks. Without these skills a child learns to talk but not to communicate. He may develop language skills, but they will not be meaningful because he will be unable to apply the language in conversational situations.

The skills include being able to make sense of facial expressions and body language, picking up helpful situational clues and ignoring those that are misleading. This is helped by the development of such things as anticipation, self-awareness, emotional understanding, and recognising the beginnings and ends of activities.

Babies are very good communicators long before they can talk, especially if given the opportunity to learn how to sign. We have seen how emotional understanding and use develops, and the importance of structure in the baby's environment to give order to a confusing world and make it easier to interpret.

◼ 'WHY ARE YOU FIXING THE PLUG, MUMMY?' ◼

TODDLER DEVELOPMENT 5

Throughout the toddler period a child accumulates understanding and knowledge of the world through observing and talking about people doing everyday things. Once she has a store of this knowledge and experience, she can try out ways of behaving and talking in different situations. These situations can range from simple shared activities like preparing a meal, to playing appropriately with friends, to negotiating conflicting expectations. A child will apply the knowledge gained through observation to help her make good sense of the situations she encounters on her own. The more experiences she has, the easier it will be for her to apply her knowledge. Before the advent of TV, children helped their mothers with everyday tasks around the family home so there were many more opportunities for them to benefit from these learning situations. Today we need to be more aware of the value of creating such opportunities.

A four- or five-year-old, when arriving at school for the first time, should have some idea of appropriate ways of engaging with a teacher – what level and type of information to give and how this is different from the way she might engage with a peer. She should also know what kind of information to give or not give a stranger. On entry to school, children should be starting to differentiate between various social situations and beginning to communicate in an appropriate style.

Within the first half-term of starting in a class, a child should be able to develop an understanding of what is expected of her and how to respond to her teacher. She should be able to recognise when the teacher is displeased, showing signs of being cross or making a joke. But many children nowadays not only don't have this skill but also don't know how to adjust their behaviour.

In this section I will talk about the development of non-verbal communication from just before the child starts talking – at any time between about one and three years. It is important to realise that, as Not Just Talking's intervention programme demonstrates, when sufficient non-verbal skills are in place speech develops naturally, and this applies regardless of the age of the child. So even in secondary school it is possible to give children who aren't talking the non-verbal conversational skills they need and, as a consequence, they will learn to talk.

The skills developed as a baby need to be refined and improved upon. The child will also have to develop new skills. In normal development the onset of talking continues to promote non-verbal skills as a by-product of the conversations she has every day. But this development depends on the child looking at the person talking to her.

In normal development all these skills develop simultaneously. I shall break them down here so that parents can be helped to identify and encourage the individual skills.

THE START OF LANGUAGE AND SPEECH

The first words

It is well documented that words start to appear singly and then are gradually put together to form phrases and sentences. This ability, although complex, is much easier for children to develop than the non-verbal communication skills. The reason for this is that it is part of normal development for parents to have a desire to hear their baby's first words. Then, on the basis of the first word, parents promote the production of other words, by pointing to other objects and saying the name – 'There's a car' or 'That's a shoe'. In time these few first words turn into two- and three-word phrases and then sentences.

Normal development of spoken language in the past was based on the assumption (which was correct although not consciously recognised) that, at the point at which the first word appears, non-verbal skills are sufficiently developed to continue alongside speech without the need for parents to give them a moment's thought. As long as the child is looking at the other person or people, she will continue to develop non-verbal skills for the rest of her life as her experience of conversational situations expands. But if this development does not occur for some reason, the skills remain at the level attained before speech began. Verbal communication skills are all present by the age of five, except for the development of vocabulary. Non-verbal communication skills keep developing for the rest of our lives. A lack of any of these skills can have a big impact on the child.

Children need opportunities to watch others communicating and to learn to decipher the clues from situations in order to ensure they develop effective non-verbal understanding. When speech takes over, it is easy for parents to assume that all is well and to promote verbal language skills without realising that the non-verbal skills are missing. When children were exposed to many more opportunities to pick up non-verbal skills every day through family mealtimes and going out to play with their peers, etc (see Palmer, 2006), development occurred more naturally. Now we need to make a conscious effort to reinforce the acquisition of non-verbal skills.

Situational understanding

When assessing and working with older children, typically eight to 14 years of age, I have frequently been struck by how little experience they have of everyday activities or the language associated with them. This may be because their behaviour is more challenging so that parents find it easier just to get on and do things quickly. Many children simply miss out on this stage of development.

Parents are also surprised when this is pointed out to them. They have assumed, as people often do when communicating with children with poor non-verbal communication skills, that they automatically understand the world in the same way as others. This is because as adults we rarely need to talk about our understanding of situations. We make an assumption that everyone knows it is time to do the washing up: we don't say 'Look at all those dirty dishes – that means we must wash up'. More likely, we will say 'You wash, I'll dry' or 'You load the dishwasher and I'll wash the saucepans', etc. We assume that the person we are talking to knows:

1 that washing up is the next activity

2 what the activity of washing up involves

3 the language associated with washing up

4 how to wash up

5 the sequence of events

6 what will happen at the end.

This understanding is only available to us if it has been stored in our subconscious from when we were very young and built upon throughout our lives. This is why elders are revered in many cultures – their experience over many years helps them to evaluate and make the right judgement about complex situations (see Section 8). Because we use this subconscious understanding every day as part of all our conversations, we don't even have to think about it. We learn by observing, analysing, doing and comparing.

As a child accumulates experiential knowledge in these formative years between the toddler and pre-school stages, she develops an understanding of everyday situations which she can apply to new and unusual settings. This 'database of information' develops in the following way:

1 Observing – watching others holding conversations.

2 Analysing – making sense of contextual clues.

3 Doing – trying out what she has observed and interpreted.

4 Comparing – assessing the response and learning what works.

Even a child who learns to talk well needs to be constantly looking at different people holding a variety of conversations. This will help her to recognise the similarities and differences between the ways people hold conversations. She will need to look at the right clues to help her store the information in her 'database'. This is the repository for all the non-verbal information that we automatically access during conversations. Her conversational skills will need to develop to allow her to ask questions or to ask for help to make better sense of what is happening, deepen her understanding and store experiences in a meaningful way for future use.

As she begins to say her first words, her parents need to make sure that she is able to expand on the non-verbal skills she has developed so far. With fewer opportunities for her to watch people holding conversations, her parents need to ensure that she is able to make the best possible use of each conversation she observes. Following the simple advice given in this book, it will be easy for them to make sure she picks up all she needs to know.

From signing to talking

As words start to appear, a toddler who has been using signs can develop the length of the signed 'phrases' she has learned to communicate with. This might occur quite suddenly because she is able to add the spoken word to her two-word signed utterances, for example, she says 'daddy' and then signs 'car' and 'home'. So from one spoken word she is able to communicate in a three-word sentence!

Gradually, as more spoken words appear and with more and more words strung together, she will drop the signing until she is only speaking. Since talking is a much more effective method of communication this will happen naturally and doesn't need encouraging. If she keeps on using the signs for longer than expected, it is because her non-verbal skills are not keeping pace with her spoken language. Parents needn't worry about the signing taking a long time to disappear. As soon as talking becomes more useful to her she will have no further need to sign.

CONVERSATIONAL LANGUAGE FUNCTIONS

The functions of language include requesting information, giving information, asking questions, etc. Children learn how to use these if given the opportunity and that may require conscious effort on the part of parents and carers. For instance, children can easily become mere receivers of information and get to school age without being able to initiate conversations effectively.

During this period a child's verbal communication skills develop markedly because in the next two or three years she will need to accumulate virtually all the skills she will need in this area for the rest of her life. The focus of this section, however, is not on verbal skill development (although in passing there may be comments about this); the focus will be how non-verbal skills develop alongside verbal language at this time. Here are some of the ways in which parents can ensure that their child can give and share information appropriately in all situations.

Naming objects, actions and people

To encourage this skill, parents should keep most of their spoken language to the level commensurate with the child's language development level. That is, when she is able to say one word the majority of comments by her parents or carers should be in the form of single words. When she has developed a range of single words and is moving towards two or more words, parents need to model two-word utterances. If they talk in longer sentences, she won't learn how to build these up for herself.

First of all, the child should start to identify what she sees: 'cat', 'dinner' 'daddy', etc. This step doesn't happen by magic but only after observing cats, for example, frequently enough to identify the features that are common to cats. This must be combined with the experience of hearing the word 'cat' whenever she sees one, repeated on many occasions by her parents/carers. Part of this process will include people pointing at the cat, even picking the cat up and letting her stroke it. The focus of the 'conversation' will be the cat – it may even be a picture (which of course will also be developing symbolisation skills).

She will also have learned by observation that eye gaze goes towards the target object or event being spoken about, but only if she has developed the interest in watching people. As a result she too will look at what is being talked about, as this is modelled. A common problem is that children often do not look at what is being spoken about and therefore cannot store and use the experience in a manner that is useful to them in other situations.

Those communicating with the child should also extend the child's speech so that she will be able to give information in two-word utterances. This is achieved by adding to the first thing that they say about the cat. This is called 'extending the utterance' and is achieved in this manner – 'Yes, it's mummy's cat' or 'It's a fat cat', and so on.

There are only two information-carrying words in these utterances and these are the ones to stress. Information-carrying words are very clearly explained in many publications on language development and intervention but are also explained well on the Cambridgeshire Community Services website (see the References).

The modelling of two-word utterances by adults or siblings also develops new types of language – verbs, adjectives, adverbs, possessive nouns, and so on. Most of the time parents do this instinctively, but frequent repetition is helpful. They should follow the advice in the previous section about identifying beginnings and endings, saying 'Bath is finished', 'Time for walk', and the like.

The use of phrases such as 'All gone!' can develop into, say, 'car gone' or 'granny gone'. The words 'bye bye' are vital at this stage as long as they have been encouraged before the baby starts to talk. Modelling 'bye bye daddy' or 'bye bye postman' or 'bye bye bricks' helps the child understand not only the two-word utterances but also the situations associated with particular words. She should notice, as long as she is looking, her parents waving at whoever is leaving and so will observe the associated body language and the common circumstance of 'going away'.

Soon, following many occasions where two-word utterances are modelled to the child, she will start to put words together, such as 'daddy gone' or 'nappy now'. These two-word utterances lead on to the child being able to extend her language functions to request information, for example.

Responding to requests

The ability to respond to a question can only be developed in a child if she is offered opportunities to do so. Parents mustn't assume that their child will pick this skill up on her own. This – and the next skill, initiation – are equally essential, but responding generally develops first.

A child needs to develop a sound understanding of the give-and-take nature of conversations. She will learn that her parents start a conversation and that she can respond, and the next step will be learning that they might reply to her response. Eventually she will start to realise that she can actually start the conversation herself.

To develop this skill her parents should ask her questions such as 'Where's teddy?' or 'Who ate the biscuit?' or 'What's daddy done?'. If the child is still not talking, she can answer using gesture, so she might point at teddy or at herself in answer to 'Who ate the biscuit?' or she might use words and say 'broken' in response to a plate being dropped.

The most important thing is that parents give the child opportunities to respond to simple conversational phrases in many different situations. Our adult tendency to predict at a high level and therefore anticipate what people want does not help to promote these skills in children.

Giving information/requesting information

The next big step for a child is to be able to initiate conversations. Many children who fail to develop this skill are misdiagnosed as being 'attention seeking'. If a child comes up to an adult and looks as though they are wanting contact but then doesn't say anything, people should ask themselves whether the child is able to initiate conversations in any other situation. She may have learned how to make contact but is unable to take it further and begin a conversation. Here is an example from a case I was involved with:

Case example

Brian was seven, in mainstream education, and in his pre-school years had had a tremendous amount of support from Portage (a home visiting service to develop skills in children with special needs), Applied Behaviour Analysis (ABA) for children on autistic spectrum and speech and language therapy, among other interventions.

When I first saw him I was told that he was 'just about to speak' as he was able to say a /b/ sound. Because everything else sounded very positive I thought that my help would not be needed. There were no behaviour issues and he was not a problem in school. However, his mother was very keen for me to see him and so I agreed to assess him and let her know what I thought.

When I arrived in his Year 2 classroom, Brian was sitting at a table with two or three other children. There was a learning support assistant sitting next to him. I observed what was happening for a few minutes. The class teacher told the assistant what she wanted the child to do, and the assistant told Brian. He did the activity then stopped. The assistant noticed that he had stopped and told this to the teacher, who then gave some more work to the assistant for the child.

I was astounded that there was no frustration in this child who couldn't respond or initiate messages apart from at a very low level. Within two weeks I had taught him to sign and he had learned so many signs that soon he was combining them.

It turned out that the reason he was unable to talk was that he had one of the severest examples of articulatory dyspraxia that I had seen as a speech and language therapist. In fact I would even call it an apraxia because on assessment at seven, despite having the biggest appetite for food and absolutely no problem at all eating, he was totally unable to open his mouth on request.

I introduced signing to Brian, a method of communication that he could use, rather than expect him to develop speech which he was a long way from achieving. Within two weeks he developed language skills and over the next few months started to give his mother so many complex messages that she could hardly keep up!

It is vital for parents to be aware of the need to develop the ability to ask for information. This is only achieved if they don't anticipate the child's needs – even if they know what the child wants for supper, they should offer her choices. They should also wait for her to ask for something, say, a book, to be passed rather than just passing the book to her. If she does this non-verbally, by holding out her hand or pointing to the book, they must respond. That is a good level of development but she also needs to practise her verbal skill of using questions and comments in a natural manner.

Some parents might feel that it is not natural to do this, but communication is no different from any other skill in as much as the way to help someone learn is not to do it for them all the time. If the child is not given the opportunity to ask for objects and activities she will not learn to initiate conversation herself. Rather than guess what the child wants, prompt her to request something, so if the child stands near the fridge the parent might assume she wants a drink. Initially, however, the parent should look at the child and communicate non-verbally 'What do you want?' Only then, if the child doesn't respond, does the parent ask the child verbally. They should try not to give the child the drink unless she has communicated in some way. This might only be to look at the door of the fridge, but at this stage this should be accepted. It is important to value the communication method used by their child. If parents ignore this attempt, it might put the child off trying again and impede the development of other ways of doing this later. Also the child might become frustrated and resort to other methods of communicating such as tantrums.

So always respond positively while the child is young if they initiate any activity or communication. Initiation is a skill that develops in many settings - it could be choosing a game and taking it to a parent or sibling to play, or offering a piece of banana to her mother.

Use of please

If the word 'please' is introduced too early before the child has learned to use a range of nouns or verbs, then 'please' becomes a magic word that does away with the need to learn more vocabulary. If you say 'please' and look at or point to something the likelihood is that you will be given it.

'Please' and 'thank you' are both words that children learn by rote from about two or three when they have a wide vocabulary, but meaning is only associated with them at a later stage – possibly as late as four or five. If the vocabulary is good, then learning these words by rote is not detrimental, but if the vocabulary is only two or three words it will seriously disadvantage the child's ability to learn more words.

'Please' and 'thank you' are merely there to make the conversation sound better socially; they are not fundamental to the message. It is better to get the communication of a child to a good level and then add the social placaters than to develop these without the child understanding what she is saying.

Asking for help

Once a child has the ability to request actions or information the next step is to be able to ask for help. Communicatively we do this all day long, mostly non-verbally – a raised eyebrow, a shrug of the shoulders, an interrogative intonation, and so on. Conversational skills improve when we help each other to understand the message.

Parents should give their child opportunities to develop this skill by encouraging the child at this age to ask for help to get drinks or do her shoes up or choose what to wear. Using non-verbal and verbal cues such as 'Do you need help?', parents can support the development of this skill so that, as she becomes more proficient in conversations, she will ask for help when she needs it.

NON-VERBAL CONVERSATIONAL SKILLS

We looked at the development of non-verbal conversational skills in babies. We are now going to look at how those skills that emerged in the first few months of life flourish during this period before the child goes to school.

There are many skills associated with conversations, but they all need to be practised over and over to ensure that when the child enters school she can communicate effectively with adults and peers. Conversations are like a game of catch (see Section 12) and therefore the child has to refine her skills as both a sender and a receiver of information.

The role of the listener

The first skill that needs to progress is that of being a good listener. There is a huge difference between listening and listener skills. You need to understand this difference in order to recognise the difficulty in children.

The role of the listener is composed of three basic elements which should be focused on first and others which, ordinarily, will develop as a natural consequence of the first three.

1   Look at the speaker.

2 Be still.

3 Listen.

The first two of these skills are the most important. As long as parents have been encouraging facial interest since the child was born they should not have to worry too much about her ability to look at the speaker. However, if the child still needs prompting to do so at this stage of development it will also be necessary to focus on why this is so. Simply telling the child to 'make eye contact' is worthless (see Section 2 on what eye contact really means). If she doesn't know why she should look at people she will not be able to interpret the non-verbal information.

Only if a child has learned to understand facial expressions and body language will looking at faces be meaningful. So parents need to go back a stage or two and develop interest in faces and understanding of what body language means. Until these skills are present it is of no benefit to the child to ask her to look at the person she is talking to. Parents and professionals should not make the assumption that she is choosing not to look or that she is merely diffident; until the age of five children have to look at people as much as possible to be proficient communicators later in their lives.

The second skill of keeping still is associated with many communication difficulties and often improves when a child is given the skills to process non-verbal information. Suffice it to say, if a child (or anyone for that matter) doesn't keep still while communicating, she won't be able to look at the person and won't be focused on picking up the message. Being fidgety or moving around too much gets in the way of taking in the non-verbal information that is vital to making good sense of what someone is saying. Moreover, the likelihood that anyone would continue to talk to a person who moved about constantly during the conversation is small and so children who do this are unlikely to maintain or keep friendships because the basic building block of friendships is conversation – see below. Fidgeting while talking to others communicates not really being interested or focused on the conversation.

The last skill in the list above is 'listen'. Now that might be self-evident and most of the children that I have worked with have some idea that being a 'good listener' is important, but have little idea what it really means in practice.

I ask the question 'How do I know you are listening?' They may be able to reel off that they need to look at the person, but generally they are unaware of the need to be still and have no idea that the key evidence that someone is listening is when they respond appropriately. The listener needs to give the information that the speaker has requested. It is no use if, when asked 'What did you have for breakfast?', the answer is 'It was snowing this morning'. The person asking the question will assume that the listener is not listening, however still or attentive they might have been. Only when we speak about the same topic or respond to a question appropriately will we be really listening. This difficulty is often called 'not sticking to topic'.

Interest in the conversation

Another vital but more demanding conversational skill that evolves at this stage is the ability to demonstrate interest in what the other person is saying. This is a really important conversational skill because it is central to a child's capacity to make and keep friends.

A child who doesn't demonstrate interest in what another child says, over time, will be less likely to be approached by other children to engage her in a conversation. We all want to know that people are interested in what we have to say – even young children. This underlines the importance of the basic give-and-take of a conversation and understanding the listener's role in keeping the conversation alive.

Giving feedback as a listener

During these toddler years, the child must also learn how to give feedback during a conversation. In normal development children go through a phase at this age of asking for endless feedback verbally. This is often through the use of the word 'why?', which can sometimes drive parents to distraction but shouldn't be stopped because it is doing two important things:

1   Giving the child experience of being able to ask for clarification in a safe and repetitive manner with their parents. (By the time she goes to school, she should have toned down her requests for clarification to be appropriate and also to include many non-verbal methods of asking for clarification.)

2   She is accumulating knowledge about the world which will be very helpful in terms of both her vocabulary and her ability to process non-verbal information in day-to-day situations, such as, 'Why are you fixing the plug, mummy?'

As we can see from the next section, a big problem for both the listener and the speaker is when they can't see the person they are speaking to.

The role of the speaker

In order to become a good speaker a child must learn about the speaker's role in the conversation. Most people assume that it is to give information and not much more than that. However, when put in a position where they can't see the listener or the listener is not giving the feedback required to keep the conversation going, then people can see that conversations are dependent on the two-way process of communication.

This is why speaking on the phone is so much more difficult. Face to face, a speaker is dependent on subtle feedback to let them know whether or not the listener is interested in and understands what they are saying – nodding, smiling, raised eyebrows, and so on. Because the other person can't be seen, we have to rely on much higher-level non-verbal communication skills such as tone of voice, intonation pattern, stress and rhythm to pick up the words to focus on, to know when it's our turn to speak, and so on. This has a big effect on both speaking and listening. On the phone it accounts for why we tend to give so much more vocal feedback, in terms of 'ah's, 'oh's, and the like, to ensure that the person talking knows they are still being listened to.

This is why trying to pick up a new language from the radio or a CD is such hard work. It is what children with poor non-verbal skills are trying to do all day long: listening to every word that is being said and trying to interpret everything equally. Our brains cannot process the spoken word at the speed at which we speak. So the brain tunes in to the important words (information-carrying words) and takes for granted the other words according to our understanding of grammatical structures and the context of the message.

My personal experience of trying to learn French this way demonstrated how difficult it was to make sense of what was being said. When listening to the radio in your mother tongue, high-level non-verbal skills direct us to the significant words. In a new language this can only be done when your verbal language is sufficiently advanced.

It is vital that children develop strengths in this area of communication. In normal development this is achieved solely through the child observing conversations that she is having or that others are having. She needs to learn how to change what she says if the listener doesn't understand or change the topic if they have had sufficient information.

Parents can point this out in a more explicit manner by saying things such as 'I didn't understand you'; 'Can you say that again please?'; 'I'm sorry but I am confused'. At the same time they need to exaggerate the facial expression that goes with this message so that the child simultaneously hears the message and sees the non-verbal expression that accompanies it. Over time she will be able to understand the message without the spoken language.

Interest in others

Conversations start from the basis that one person is sufficiently interested in the other to share information with them. This skill grows from those early attempts to get babies interested in faces. They learn that people are interesting and do unusual things that are worth enquiring about.

Interest in people can be expanded in these toddler years if parents or childminders help the child to participate in different activities, such as reading books and playing games, in different social settings such as playgroups, mother and toddler groups, with childminders, parties, other family homes, and so on. The more the child is keen to make contact with other people the more likely she is to want to communicate with them.

In the first few months of life a baby learns to distinguish close relatives from those people she doesn't know so well. This ability to recognise similarities and differences in people's faces now needs to deepen and expand so that she gets a real understanding of those people in her friendship group and those who are strangers. There is a great deal to say about this skill and the consequences of failure to develop it.

87

Styles

Styles of conversation change according to who the other person is and the situation in which the conversation is taking place. So we would talk in one way to a vicar in a church – which would affect not only the content and style but the volume of speech as well – and in another way to a friend in the pub. There are different styles for conversations at home and at work, in hospital or the police station, at the supermarket or in a haute couture shop. We adjust all day long using our non-verbal interpretation of the person and the situation alongside our past experience of similar situations. Most of the time as adults we get this right but, even then, it is easy to get it wrong sometimes.

The ability to interpret a wide variety of circumstances and situations is key. Children need to have observed many different styles of conversations among people of different ages – not only at home but at the doctor's, library, baker's shop, a friend's house. If a child has seen only one style modelled then she will learn to talk only in that style, which will be inappropriate in many situations.

Rules

This section refers to the unspoken 'rules' we apply to many different situations and specifically those rules that make a conversation work. In every situation a toddler needs to apply or test out a rule that she has observed others using. This testing out is to ascertain whether she has recognised correctly the similarities between two different situations. For example, if her mother tells her not to stand so close when she is talking to her, the next time she talks to her mother she will try standing in a different position. If this gets a positive response she will then stand that distance away from others to see if they respond positively as well.

If she notices that, when her father is talking to her mother, her mother is not talking at the same time, the child tries not talking at the same time as others. If this gets a good reaction from her parents, the rule becomes confirmed and validated. It is very important for parents to notice when she has applied a rule correctly and praise her, so they could say 'Good getting ready for dinner' or 'Good sitting still', depending on the activity.

Whenever we go into situations as adults we apply unspoken rules about how to behave in that situation. For example, when attending a training session participants know from previous experience to sit and listen to the person who is deemed to be the 'trainer' and not to fire a barrage of questions at them before the subject has even been introduced. If parents have been developing all the precursor non-verbal skills necessary, then they should only have to encourage and monitor their child in applying the correct rules to situations.

Making friends

As with most of the things that we do all day, such as deciding on the day's activities over breakfast, talking to the postman, ringing the doctor, choosing which TV programme to watch, and so forth, we depend on conversations to make satisfactory choices and get things done. Making and keeping friends is also totally dependent on conversational skills. There is a great difference in skill between making friends and keeping friends. Both require good conversational skills; but keeping friends needs much better ones.

To make friends a child might go up to another child and tell them what she is interested in or ask them to join in a game. Quite quickly a friendship may develop, as long as the other party is interested in what the first child wants to do. Many children with non-verbal communication problems can do this part of the friendship building because they can talk about what interests them and initially appear very knowledgeable and fascinating.

However, the next stage of keeping the friendship going depends on the child having good understanding of the role of both speaker and listener. Not only do they need to give information but they have to share information too. This means being able to ask the other person for information about their likes and dislikes. The children I have worked with find this really hard before the intervention. They want to dominate the conversation so that they won't be asked questions that they cannot answer.

Sharing information involves not only asking what your conversational partner likes but also giving information about your interest in that topic. Here are two conversations, one of which is sharing information and the other is not:

Fred: 'I have this amazing game of fantasy that is about a boy who meets a wizard and they go to a forest and in the forest the wizard gives the boy some magic powers. The boy can run like the wind and turn anything into what he wants it to be. I like this game and I have decided to develop it into a computer programme so that I can play it on my computer and then you can play it on your computer too.'

Mark: 'What's it called?'

Fred: 'The boy then goes home to see his mum and she says "Where have you been?", but the boy runs upstairs to try out his powers …' etc.

Here is a second version of the same conversation:

Fred: 'Hi Mark, guess what? I have developed a really good game. Would you like to hear about it?'

Mark: 'Yes, what happens?'

Fred: 'It's about a boy who goes into a wood and meets a wizard. He gives the boy special powers.'

Mark: 'What powers are they?'

Fred: 'He can run like the wind and turn anything into what he needs it to be but for only one day. Have you played a game like that before?'

Mark: 'I think so but the boy became a wizard too.'

Fred: 'Well, I think that one sounds interesting, I'll see if I can make my boy into a wizard too.'

In the first conversation, Fred is giving all the information and doesn't pay any attention to what Mark says. He also just carries on giving information, not leaving opportunities for his friend to ask anything. This is not sharing information at all, it is just giving information.

In the second conversation, Fred is pausing in what he says. This is to give Mark an opportunity to ask or say something. Fred then responds to what Mark has said before adding other information that he might not know.

Children who can't share information want to tell you what they may know about their favourite subject because they are confident talking about this topic. We all like to do this, but with good conversational skills we generally develop the ability to talk about more than one or two favourite subjects! Other children, having at first been fascinated by what the child is saying, soon become fed up with the lack of two-way traffic in the conversation and also feel that the child is not really interested in talking to them because they don't look at them when talking (see 'The role of the listener' above).

So the child can start up a friendship but it doesn't develop or last. If this happens over and over again, the child can become confused (because she doesn't understand why it is happening) or depressed because she can't make friends. Children I have worked with are desperate to make friends but just don't know how to make things work better.

So children must learn how to share information. This happens early on as conversations develop. The more they can practise this the more their interest in others will develop. Then they will start asking for information to find out what others think, feel or want to do, developing more areas of shared interest. If this skill is developing naturally there is nothing to worry about, but parents whose toddlers are not learning how to share information with people should make sure that they learn to do so before entering school.

Complexity of groups and interactive speaking

During this period of being a toddler and developing all these essential conversational skills, a child will go from being able to talk to one person at a time – their parent, sibling or carer – to being able to talk in small groups and then larger groups. This development is an essential step that the child needs to make before entry to school. Without the ability to cope with groups the child will find life at school intolerable.

INTERPRETATIONAL SKILLS

This section is all about the further development in the understanding and use of facial expressions and body language. Before a child enters school, she must look at many faces (and witness many conversations) in all sorts of different situations – by this stage the quantity should be in the hundreds if not the thousands.

The number of faces she sees is very important so that she is able to compare and contrast the similarities and differences between them all. Then she will be able to make progress in understanding the more advanced facial expressions and body language.

Boundaries

Throughout the toddler phase of development the child must continue to learn about the sometimes quite low-key signals that communicate the start and finish of activities. Parents need to tell the child what they are going to do, and talk about the process of the activity and the end of the activity, for instance, making cakes. The parent says, 'We are going to make some cakes. First we need to mix the cakes then cook them in the oven and then we can eat them. Let's start with a mixing bowl.' Then, while each part of the process happens, they will talk about what they are doing. At the end they can say, 'Cooking is finished. Now it's time to eat the cakes!'

By doing this for every activity, parents will ensure that the child is picking up the signals for the start and finish of activities, which in time will evolve into recognising boundaries of all kinds. Without the skill to process this information, a child will be unable to recognise clear boundaries set by parents about what type of behaviours are acceptable and which are not as she grows older. Children who cannot identify boundaries are more likely to display tantrum behaviour for a longer period of time than is usually expected.

Tantrums

Tantrums usually develop for a short period when the child is about two years old. This is why people refer to the 'terrible twos'. The reason for this period of tantrum behaviour is because the child's spoken language skill outstrips her non-verbal communication skills for a short period. The child is able to speak better but is unable to process the spoken word at the speed of her speech. Temporarily, her ability to interpret and predict from the non-verbal information available is lagging behind her other communication skills.

Therefore, in a situation that is tedious or demanding for her, such as being out shopping for a long time or being asked to do something at home that she doesn't want to do, she doesn't have the words she needs so resorts to tantrum behaviour. This includes screaming and shouting, kicking and hitting out. Read about the strategies adopted by older children in the section about problems associated with poor non-verbal communication, you will see the similarity in the behaviours!

The period of tantrums is also extended if the child is unable to recognise signals which indicate the beginning and end of activities. The introduction of signs at the baby stage will help tremendously as the child will be able to use the signs to support her communication when her verbal language lets her down. So if parents develop these skills well in their child, the tantrum period should be brief.

Emotional understanding

As we have seen, a baby's level of emotional understanding is quite basic, recognising only simple, clear or vivid emotional states. Now that the child is learning to talk this understanding has to make a huge leap forward. The evidence she is observing becomes less overt and more low-key as situations multiply and facial expressions become more muted. So it requires much more attention to people's faces and she will need a lot of help from her parents to develop her awareness of clues. Parents are only likely to draw her attention to this more subtle information if they are aware of the need to help her.

Levels of emotional understanding

The child needs to be able to recognise emotions at a mid-level now, such as a face that is content or satisfied rather than exaggeratedly happy, as she will see in normal, everyday communication. Because the clues are less clear cut, she will need to be more attentive to faces even when she is not involved in the conversation. These times are almost as important as one-to-one interactions she has because she should be seeing two (or more) people making these lower-level expressions.

This leads to another key skill area she will need to develop before school. Not only does she need to recognise different facial expressions in her parents or carers and siblings, but she also has to recognise the same expressions in other people with whom she is less familiar. We all communicate through facial expressions in a similar but slightly different manner.

So, for example, the child must learn to notice that, when Mrs Brown, the neighbour, is moderately happy she shows it in a similar manner to mummy, that is, she smiles but not too much and her eyes widen a bit, but unlike mummy she doesn't nod her head at the same time. Apply this simple example to more complex situations and the importance of recognising similarity and difference will become clear. Here are some examples of people who communicate irritation in slightly different ways:

- Father: makes a frown combined with a quizzical look. He may also raise a hand with a pointed finger. He uses a sing-song, slightly sarcastic, stern voice.

- Mother: makes a frown but purses her lips; her body tenses a little and she puts her hands on her hips.

- Teacher in primary school: frowns a bit, makes her voice deeper and more formal, her body becomes straight and slightly tense and she looks disapprovingly at the individual or group causing the problem.

- Friends: can do this in a variety of ways – stamping, throwing things, walking away. And some may have non-verbal communication problems and therefore don't show irritation at all or do so in an idiosyncratic manner.

- Teachers in secondary school: the problem is highly exacerbated in secondary education as the child then has to see and make sense of a number of different teachers in a day, some of whom might not be seen more than once in the week! If added up it could reach more than 10 teachers per week, plus others such as Head,

 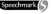

Deputy, Head of tutorial group, SENCO, dinner staff, and the rest.

The variation in the above five examples alone could be very confusing to a child who has not developed the ability to recognise the variety of emotional expression.

Notice also the huge shift from primary to secondary school in the number of faces that a child will have to look at and understand. This is the explanation (when added to other social and educational pressures on children at secondary school) for the high referral rate to Not Just Talking of children in their first year at secondary school.

Toddlers who don't develop these complex skills and who can't process non-verbal information in the manner described here are very vulnerable as teenagers because they do not pick up the clues telling them either not to do something or to get out of the way of trouble. This is why it is vital that, having learned to recognise basic emotions, the child develops the awareness that others communicate similar emotions in ways that might be a bit different but mean the same thing. Then she needs to be able to compare and differentiate in order to interpret accurately.

By the time she enters school she should, at the very least, be able to identify in her parents low, mid- and high-level emotional communication in more than 10 emotions, such as happy, angry, bored, loving, sad, surprised, and so on. Different children may learn different emotions; it is more about the number and range of different emotions, both positive and negative.

Understanding family relationships

This is an extremely complex area of development, but the foundations are laid during the toddler years and will be really necessary in her later years. The key is to understand that people can have relationships with people other than herself and that this does not affect the relationship a person has with her.

A child has to develop relationships with her mother and father. The roles are very different, as the mother's role is to give the child love and attention while the father's role is to help the child understand that she is able to have more relationships and that they will be different. In single parent families, if there isn't another person with whom the child can develop a relationship that is not the 'mothering' relationship, she will find relating to other people much harder. This can be overcome by ensuring that the child has regular contact with a significant other – grandmother or uncle. But it has to be someone with a different type of relationship with the child. It won't work if this person mothers the child too.

So the child learns from the non-verbal clues what her relationship with her mother is and how it differs from that with her father. She should also start to appreciate that her parents' love for her is constant and although at times they might be angry with her, this underlying relationship is not affected. Parents need to be aware of the importance of their child learning this skill, before she enters school.

Singletons may also find this harder as they are unable to develop the skills associated with sharing your parents with your siblings. But as with all these 'problem' areas for non-verbal communication development, as long as people are aware of the importance of exposure to different relationships, then the child will develop the ability.

Direction of movement

It might seem strange, but we need to learn what direction of movement tells us. We are not born knowing that if people are walking away from us and we can see their backs, they are moving away, or if we can see their front then they are more likely to be coming towards us. This needs to be applied at a basic level before it can be understood in more complex circumstances, such as whether a queue of children is queuing to go out of the class or come back into the class.

Body tension

As we have already seen, muscle tension or relaxation communicates a great deal non-verbally. Think about what tension communicates (anger, fear, excitement) and how a relaxed body or arm communicates different things. For example, when we observe someone standing loosely with their head bowed and arms not tensed, it is easy to conclude that the person is likely to be sad. The degree of tension a person exhibits helps you decide whether you should approach them or avoid them.

It is important for a child to be able to pick up this information from the tension or relaxation of bodies when looking at people. It will tell her whether the person is cross and demanding that the child look at something or simply pointing out something of interest to the child. The child will be more likely to communicate appropriately if she has interpreted this effectively. This absence or use of tension can be identified from the back view of people or from far away before the child is able to hear what the person is saying. So the child could take avoiding action if necessary.

If a child is unable to pick up these signals she will be very vulnerable to finding herself in conflict situations that she will be unable to negotiate her way out of.

Body language use

A toddler continues to develop as she did as a baby, that is to say, understanding of the levels of emotions comes before the ability to use them. So once the child has learned to recognise different levels of emotions and the causes of these emotions in others, she can begin to apply the associated facial expressions and body language in similar situations.

Children will only use body language and facial expressions that they have seen and learned. So parents need to be aware that, just as their child will experiment by copying simple words or gestures, so she is trying out and using the more sophisticated body language associated with emotions.

As we have seen, nursery rhymes and action songs are central to the development of gesture and body language and therefore are a central part of how a child will learn to be a good communicator in all its aspects.

Touch

Another important non-verbal skill that needs to develop easily during this toddler phase is the knowledge about who it is and is not acceptable to touch and how to touch people appropriately depending on the person and situation. This ranges from the early cuddles and hugs that parents give their children to situations where it might be appropriate to hug another person who isn't a family member; for example, if another child hurt themselves while playing, a toddler might go and show sympathy and support with a hug.

Before school entry children must begin to understand that hugging a teacher or dinner lady is not appropriate and that hugging strangers is definitely out of the question. Again this is all dependent upon her ability to recognise and process non-verbal information telling her who is a close friend and who is a stranger – see 'Interest in others' above.

There are a few aspects concerning touch that parents should make sure that their child is aware of before school entry, including:

- appropriate and inappropriate kinds of touching – squeezing, pinching, hitting, stroking, hugging, etc

- touching with fingers, hands or other parts of the body

- where on other people's bodies it is permitted to touch

- situational rules about touching different parts of her own body.

All this needs to be learned and will only be learned if the toddler sees others touching and parents commenting about what the different types of touch mean. Nursery rhymes can play a big role in the development of this understanding because of all the movement, touching and repetition involved, for example in 'Incy Wincy Spider', ' Ten in a bed', 'Knock at the door', 'Ten fat sausages'. If a child is having a problem with touch then make up rhymes where different types of touch are involved, such as gentle, tickling, loving, and so on.

Proximity

Proximity means knowing how close to get to people. Again, this is based on our understanding of the person and the situation, so all the skills talked about in this book are the foundation for applying awareness of proximity appropriately.

Toddlers learn about proximity through experience – as when the child stands too close and her parent says 'I don't want you to stand so close to me' (or words to that effect). The toddler will then move and if the parent doesn't repeat the phrase or says something like 'That's right' to confirm that the distance chosen is suitable, then next time the child is in a similar situation she will be encouraged to test out her 'rule' to see if it applies.

Parents should not assume that, when they tell their child not to do something, the child knows what the rule is that she should be using for this particular situation. So it is always best if they say, 'I don't want you to stand so close. I want you to stand there' and indicate where with their hand.

Situations

All the above information will also help a child to interpret situations better. She needs to learn to focus on the signs within situations that are helpful and to ignore all those that are not useful to her communicatively. So throughout her toddler years parents should help her to focus on the meaningful indicators so that she can make good sense of what is happening.

A child needs to start accumulating rules that work and recognising those that don't work. These will tell her what is expected so that she can start to apply the behaviours and rules that are applicable in different situations. The foundation of these is interpretational skills. Unless she identifies signals that carry meaning and gets the interpretation right, she won't be able to speculate on the appropriate communication or behaviour for the situation. This will be so important for her later use of this skill in secondary school.

COGNITIVE SKILLS

Recognising similarities and differences

Parents should talk to their children from a very early age about the similarities and differences between objects, events, animals, people, and so on. The more chances children have to develop the skill of identifying similarities and differences and to apply this knowledge to situations and people, the more likely they are to be able to recognise people they know and those they don't. Desmond Morris, author of important books on human behaviour such as Manwatching and The Naked Ape (1997, 1969), points out how people look at each other when passing, just to establish with the briefest of glances whether the person is in their store of known people.

This skill doesn't magically appear overnight. It must be developed and honed over the period before a child reaches her teenage years. So as long as the child has been through the development spoken about in Section 4 and is able to recognise that she is a separate entity, she can go on to refine her awareness of those people she knows well, those she knows slightly and those she doesn't know at all.

This leads on to knowing what to say to people and helps her develop an understanding of shared knowledge (see below).

Connecting information

After a toddler has developed the skill of making good sense of situations, she then has to be able to connect information gained in one situation that might be helpful in another. This ability to associate and compare situational information is an important step in accurate interpretation, and it is very obvious when the child is unable to do this.

Parents need to ensure their child is able to use information such as 'granny likes blue flowers' in another situation. So, for instance, when the child is drawing some flowers she might make them blue, perhaps including granny in the picture – connecting 'granny', 'blue' and 'flowers'. Another example of this is to remember when a friend wants to be called by a nickname instead of their real name, connecting the visual clue of the friend with the nickname and the knowledge that being called this name pleases the friend. Applying information of this kind in simple and more complex situations is a vital communication skill that will help her to say or do the right thing and develop successful relationships.

The skill is built on parents talking about what they see and what they are doing in everyday situations so that the child can associate clues relating to particular circumstances or activities – washing clothes, feeding the ducks or making sandwiches. By looking and listening, the child will gather information so that when she goes to her friend's house she will be able to associate the common features that help her to recognise 'bathroom', 'playhouse', 'mealtime', and so on. She is also accumulating new vocabulary to apply in these situations.

On assessment children often can't make these connections, but intervention enables them not only to connect the information but also to apply it appropriately – even those on the autistic spectrum.

Symbolic understanding

Most professionals working within the field of child development will know about this area of development, so this is just a summary of the stages from the perspective of non-verbal communication skill development.

A symbol stands for the object or action it relates to. It may be an image, an object or a sound. The development of symbolic understanding starts in the first year of life and continues until the child is fully talking. The spoken word is the most difficult to achieve as the experience of hearing a word is so fleeting. The written word develops after the spoken word, usually once the child has entered school, and can be viewed over time to help make sense of it.

In order to attain full symbolic understanding, the child will need to pass through the earlier levels. The levels of symbolisation I have promoted with pre-verbal children are:

1   real objects

2   reduced-size objects, such as a tea-set for a doll

3   photos of objects

4   drawings of objects

5   miniature objects

6   symbols

7   spoken word

8   written word.

It is not possible for a child to skip the first five levels, although some might develop concurrently, so the understanding of symbols (such as those on road signs) might develop alongside the spoken word. A child needs to be competent at symbolisation for verbal communication to develop. Children with non-verbal communication difficulties who are able to speak will demonstrate good symbolic understanding.

But non-verbal children, such as those with autism, need help to move up the levels. Progression won't happen until the child is competent at the previous level of symbolic development. They may also need a longer period of consolidation at the individual levels.

Shared knowledge

Shared knowledge refers to that knowledge that is common to a group of people, for example, a family. Within families there is a great deal of knowledge about what members of the family do. This can range from daddy and/or mummy going to work, to Friday night being swimming night, to the eldest son's name being Peter and a huge amount of other detail about relationships, activities and experience.

All this shared understanding avoids the need to describe each person and situation before getting to the nub of the utterance: it allows a kind of verbal shorthand. So instead of saying:

> *When we go swimming before tea on Friday, we will need our swimming costumes and towels. Shall we call your friend Sadie to see if she wants to come too?*

the parent or carer could say:

> *Shall we call Sadie and see if she wants to go with us on Friday?*

The fact that on Friday the family go swimming before tea is shared knowledge and doesn't have to be stated, as is the fact that swimming involves costumes and towels, so that can be left out too. The speaker also knows that the child has a friend called Sadie. The only new bit of information is about whether or not Sadie is going to come.

However, when communicating with people outside the group or family, the situation is quite different. When she goes into class on a Monday morning the child may be asked by the teacher, 'What did you do at the weekend?' The child needs to know that the teacher was not there with her at the weekend and does not have shared knowledge of the family, therefore she will have to give more contextual information in her reply:

We went with Sadie on Friday. It was great

doesn't give the teacher enough context to understand what the girl is saying. The teacher would have to ask supplementary questions, and probably more than one or two, to get the information she was really seeking. What the girl said in this instance would have been appropriate if she had been talking to her parents or siblings because they would have known what had happened on Friday. The girl needs to say something like this to help her teacher know what she is talking about:

On Friday we went to pick my friend Sadie up to go swimming in Worcester. Afterwards we all went bowling. We had a great time.

Now there is sufficient information to let the teacher know what happened, and if the teacher wants to know more she can ask supplementary questions.

Quantity of information

Knowing how much information to give people and getting it right is a difficult skill that takes years of practice to achieve. Too little information leaves the listener dissatisfied but too much information overloads them. Getting it right is a combination of many skills, including interpretation and shared knowledge.

The foundation of appropriate levels of information is in shared knowledge – an understanding of what your listener may or may not know about the topic. For instance, a child should know that when she talks to her friend about the trip they both made to the zoo, she won't need to be very explicit as the friend will have a lot of the same information in her head. However, if she tells a friend who didn't go on the trip, she will have to give enough detail to help this friend understand what happened. She will also have to keep looking at her listener to make sure that they are still interested in what she is saying. Otherwise she will overload her listener and may put them off talking to her in future.

By now a toddler should be looking at her listener and be able to recognise a face that tells her the listener is really interested in what she is saying or has heard enough on that topic. Parents need to observe whether this is happening day-to-day and should help her out if she overloads people by pointing out these signals and telling her what they mean. Soon the child should only need to be prompted by the use of phrases such as, 'That's enough about your new book, Molly'.

Change

Difficulties in dealing with change are widely recognised in many children, particularly those on the autistic spectrum. Many establishments make effective use of visual clues to support these children. However, by ensuring that an understanding of change develops in the first place, or developing it if it is not present using Not Just Talking intervention techniques, these children become less dependent on visual clues.

Parents need to help their child recognise the signals that indicate change is about to happen. Developmentally, children do this between about two and four years of age. The best way that parents can ensure that their child notices change is to start by making bold signals for positive changes. They should also check that the child knows how to deal with good changes before introducing any that might be emotionally challenging, for instance, 'We can't go to the park, so let's go swimming instead.'

The child will soon need to recognise more complex or subtle signals of change such as her mother getting the car keys out – indicating that they will be going in the car. This is particularly important before she enters school. The child's level of understanding depends on parents having followed the recommendation to signal the start and finish of all activities during the baby period of development. As long as parents have been drawing their child's attention to these clues, they will not need to mark changes for very long. Parents should just say something like, 'Oh dear, we can't go to play at David's house so let's play football instead.' However, if the child has not developed this skill of recognising the beginnings and ends of activities, parents will need to continue to support their child by keeping the signals bold and explicit for a longer period.

The really important things to remember are to:

- be clear about the nature of the change

- offer an alternative if possible

- make the change no less interesting to the child than the activity that can't be done.

At the same time, parents should associate an exaggerated intonation pattern and arm movements with the 'Oh dear' part of the message so that the child will have more clues to draw on than just the words. This will make it more likely that the message will be stored and used in other situations.

Once parents are certain that their child understands examples of positive change, they can then introduce the use of 'Oh dear!' with a negative type of change: 'Oh dear, we can't go to the swings, let's go to the supermarket instead', or 'Oh dear, we can't go and see granny, let's make the beds instead' – something the child won't have chosen to do.

Once parents are sure that their child is able to recognise different types of change and react to them in a positive manner they can be sure that their child will cope at school more readily.

What is choice and how does it develop?

The capacity to deal with choice is a central skill for communication on many levels. Choosing requires communication, so it allows a child to practise her conversational skills. Without choice the child is automatically given things and has no need to communicate.

First we need to look at the development of the skill of choosing.

1 Make sure that the choices are offered at the correct symbolic level: real objects, small objects, photos, symbol or written word.

2 Offer choices clearly – one choice in each hand. Keep the choices clearly separated so that if she just looks to indicate her choice, it is evident which one she is choosing.

3 Use small trays if the child is finding it hard – put the choices on two trays. This gives a frame round the objects that some children find helpful.

4 It is important for parents to start by offering a positive and a negative choice, so, for example, a pudding choice should include one that the child definitely wouldn't want to eat. Giving a choice of two things the child likes does not allow parents to identify that she has made an active choice.

5 Parents should be aware how easy it is to think that their child is choosing when she is not. She may have just learned the procedure and knows that her parents want her to take one of the items. If choice has not been developed in the manner described in (1) then the child won't be able to apply this skill to other situations.

6 Then parents can develop this into a choice between two puddings (or other items) she likes because they now know she can choose.

7 Choosing must include an option for the child to reject the choices offered, otherwise it is not a genuine choice.

8 Signalling the choice or rejection of choice, combined with signs for choosing and rejection, is a good method of establishing this skill: 'You have chosen the yoghurt. You don't want the banana.'

9 A possible sign for choice is to curl up the three middle fingers to your palm and point the thumb and little finger towards the object chosen, saying 'Choose', and when she has chosen, 'Good choosing'. The sign for rejection is to make a 'pushing away' movement from the stomach with the back of the hand towards the body (thumb downward). Parents can use another sign as long as the same sign is used consistently to mean 'no'.

Once the skill is established, parents can offer many choices throughout the day to ensure that their child is honing this skill and will be able to make informed choices later in life.

Because the activity of choosing also offers opportunities to practise asking for information, clarification or help as well as giving information, it is a wonderful way of helping children to exercise their conversational skills.

Prediction

We looked at the importance of this skill for communication in Section 4, and as the child becomes older the ability to predict is increasingly crucial. In order to communicate effectively it is vital that we are able to predict the following information in conversations:

1 What the topic of conversation is about.

2 What the other person might know about the topic.

3 What and how much they might need or want to know.

4 What their reaction to the conversation might be – if they were going to be upset by it, this might determine what should be said to avoid making matters worse.

To develop their child's ability to predict, parents need to model their own understanding by commenting on situations they observe together, for instance, 'Look, that man is going to get on his bike and ride it.'

Only when the child is showing evidence of being able to predict should parents introduce the next stage of development and ask something like, 'Look at that man. What do you think he is going to do?' If the child can't do this, then the parent should model what the child could say by saying something along the lines of, 'He has his helmet on; I see him holding the handlebars and that makes me think he is going to get on the bike and ride it.'

This type of question must be applied in all situations relating to single people and groups of people. It should encompass not only what the people are going to do, as in the example above, but also what they are likely to be talking about (prompt the child to give both sides of the conversation) as well as what they might be thinking and feeling.

The other aspect of prediction that will affect the child's communication is that it enables us to know what is likely to happen to us and therefore reduces our levels of anxiety. We all communicate much more easily when feeling confident and it is virtually impossible to feel confident if we are anxious. Remember that this skill of prediction helps the child to recognise that things happen in sequence.

Parents should not ignore opportunities to ensure that their child can predict in all senses of the word. These are excellent opportunities for reinforcing other conversational skills as well.

Speculation

The ability to speculate leads on from choice and prediction and therefore is important in helping the child to find the right thing to do and say. We subconsciously evaluate any situation by processing the non-verbal signals from the people present, reading clues from the situation or context and comparing our experience of similar circumstances.

Our behaviour is based on our assessment of this information, and whether or not we behave appropriately depends on how accurate the assessment is. The ability to consider options and alternatives, to speculate about possible scenarios, helps us refine our choices and select appropriate behaviour for the situation.

In my experience this ability to speculate is poorly developed in many children. Consequently, when asked what they think is going on in a situation they often come up with a completely unexpected answer. Here is an example of what can happen to children if it goes wrong.

> *When shown a picture of two young children waiting in the reception area of a swimming pool I have often been told that these people are in a garden centre. This is because the children have focused on one clue – the reception area has a large pot plant in it despite two other very obvious clues – the children carrying rolled-up towels and their mother paying for tickets at reception.*

When asked, after coming to the wrong conclusion about this situation, what else might be going on, the children are often unable to even attempt a guess. They can only think of one option. In a conversational situation we have to be able to keep on speculating as we piece together the evidence until we come to the correct conclusion about the situation. Then we can adjust our behaviour accordingly. If a child hasn't developed the skill of analysis and speculation based on what she can see, she will be limited to what might be a false understanding of the situation.

Confidence and self-esteem

If we are on top of our subject and also confident that our communication skills will not let us down, we will become better communicators. So it is vital that children become confident in their communication skills. They can do this as long as they are able to predict effectively and have knowledge of their topic.

Children on the autistic spectrum may appear to be confident because they talk readily and fluently about their favourite topics. But if asked to talk about something else or placed in an unfamiliar situation their confidence can evaporate. Confidence needs to be present in most situations to make us good communicators.

Virtually all the 300-plus children I have worked with over the past 15 years on assessment were found to be lacking in self-esteem. But all of them improved significantly in this area following intervention and as a result of having good conversational skills – including the ability to predict – on which they could depend. By ensuring that these skills develop adequately in the toddler years, we can enable the child to enter school confidently and feel really good about themselves.

Conflict and negotiation

In order to deal with conflict, a child first of all needs to be able to process the non-verbal information in a situation and come up with more than one option of how to behave. But if the child has that skill and there is still conflict, then the child must also know how to negotiate her way out of trouble.

This ability to negotiate is a very high-level conversational skill which children going into school are just learning to do. Toddlers (two to four years) do not have sufficient skills and should always be helped to negotiate, especially with other children, when the situation deteriorates. It is through modelling of this high-level conversational skill that children learn over time how to do it for themselves. For example, when finding the child in an argument or another position where negotiation is required, the adult should step in and negotiate on her behalf if she hasn't developed the skill. Then afterwards they should talk through how the conversation went, what was said to make things better and how the other person reacted. Opportunities to observe this over time will help her develop the skills for herself.

If the child finds this really hard, parents could try this approach:

Use toys to model this conversation. Tell the child that teddy and dolly want to play a game. Teddy wants to play cars and dolly wants to play tea parties. Talk about how they could negotiate and then act out the situation.

If the child has no idea how to do this, model it for her. Parents need to give the child the skill to take control of the negotiation. Help her negotiate in positive situations and then she will be able to develop the skills for the more complex situations where conflict is involved.

Drawing conclusions

The ability to draw conclusions from visual information is fundamental to communication. A child who can't do this is only able to describe what she can see, that is, 'The man is sitting on a chair and the girl is reading a book, the rest of the books are on the shelves' rather than 'They are in a library'. It is this ability to draw a conclusion that allows us to go straight to the nub of the conversation.

If we had to elaborate all the time as in the example above, then conversations would take far too long and people would give up. It is therefore important that parents know that their child is able to do this and not assume that she can automatically formulate a conclusion.

At school, it will be expected that she has this skill because teachers will want her to be able to draw inferences and conclusions from what she has read. Without this basic skill she will be unable to get the most out of reading and learning.

Parents need to model how they draw conclusions if their child only describes things, for instance, in the example above they might say, 'Where are they?' or 'Yes, they are in the library'. Encourage the child to give this type of information first. But parents must remember that this ability to infer only develops after the skills associated with complex interpretation – shared knowledge, prediction, interpretation, and so on.

Theory of mind

Theory of mind is the ability to attribute mental states, beliefs, intentions and so forth to others – its absence is a central part of autistic spectrum disorders, that is, those diagnosed with autistic spectrum disorders are unable to do this. Theory of mind and how it relates to the Not Just Talking's work with children with poor non-verbal communication is covered in Section 12.

As Baron-Cohen and colleagues (1985) have pointed out, theory of mind starts to develop within the first year of life. Being able to interpret what people are feeling and thinking is a basic communication skill which leads on to the child being able to predict what a conversation is about and therefore give information of a useful nature.

I believe that theory of mind is central to communication itself; that the failure to develop it is not peculiar to autism and that it is therefore possible to develop this skill in many children who show signs of lacking theory of mind. But at this toddler stage of development, parents just need to ensure that they are always commenting about what they are thinking or what others might be thinking: 'I am feeling really tired because I have worked hard cleaning the car' or 'That man is asking his wife what she wants to eat', and asking the child questions such as: 'What is that boy doing? Why is he doing it?'; 'What are those children talking about?'; 'What are those children going to do?'

Anything that gets the child to put herself in someone else's shoes and see the world from their perspective will help establish these skills. But if this is not done from an early age she will not accumulate the understanding required for everyday communication.

RESOURCES

Nursery rhymes

As we saw in Section 4, nursery rhymes are a valuable tool for promoting many non-verbal and verbal skills. At this age parents need to continue to use nursery rhymes daily, as the repetition will particularly help with the high-level non-verbal skills to do with recognition of intonation, stress and rhythm patterns, all of which are fundamental to helping us know which words carry meaning and which we can ignore.

Also, children's predictive skills develop as they become interested in the more complicated nursery rhymes, such as 'Jack and Jill', 'London's Burning', 'I'm a little teapot'. This is because these longer rhymes have more opportunities for the child to fill in the next line or lines.

As the child grows older she can join in action songs which help reinforce many non-verbal skills. The simple repetition of these rhymes is a fun and effective way of developing the skills of prediction, anticipation, use and understanding of intonation, rhythm, volume, rate and stress.

The sing-song intonation of the rhymes helps the child to acquire the 'English' language intonation pattern at the root of all their spoken communication. Otherwise children can end up talking in a monotonous voice, unaware of how to use intonation or what meaning can be gained from it. Popular or traditional games based on rhymes are also good for prediction and anticipation, for instance 'Oranges and lemons'.

Here are a few examples of traditional rhymes that achieve all these things (Williams & Beck, 1987):

1 'Two fat gentlemen' – this rhyme is particularly good for getting children to understand the different styles of conversations. It starts off saying, 'Two fat gentlemen met in the lane, bowed most politely and bowed once again. How do you do? How do you do? And how do you do once again?' This is repeated four times for: two fine ladies; two tall policemen; two young schoolboys and two babies. Each time the rhymes can be said in the type of voices that would be used, so the policemen might say in an exaggerated 'policeman'-type way, 'Hello, hello, hello'!

2 'Oranges and lemons' – this rhyme also shows the development of speed of speech. It is important to know when and where to speak slowly or fast. The situation and the people tell us when this is necessary, so practising it in this way through a group game helps to develop a difficult skill. At the start of the rhyme the words are said at normal speed, but as it gets to the part that says 'Here comes a candle to light you to bed, here comes the chopper to chop off your head, chip chop, chip chop, the last man's dead', the speed increases as the children pass under the bridge made by two adults until the bridge comes down and catches one child. The simple act of doing this nursery rhyme can help the child to know that speeded-up speech suggests that something is going to happen and that slower speech is the everyday way we talk.

3 'The wheels on the bus' – good repetition with body movements and kids really love it. They will have to look closely to pick up the movements and the repetition encourages prediction.

Remember that the other areas that nursery rhymes help with are facial interest and speaker and listener skills. Knowing when it is your turn to add the next phrase is also developed.

Another non-verbal communication skill that nursery rhymes really help to develop is understanding the signals for beginnings and ends. The exaggerated stress and intonation patterns help the child know when the line or phrase is going to end, for example:

> Hickory dickory dock
> The mouse ran up the clock!
> The clock struck one
> The mouse ran down
> Hickory dickory dock.

This emphasis on the ends of the lines helps draw attention to stress and intonation patterns which in a complex way signal much to do with many aspects of communication. These are difficult aspects of communication both to understand and to use, but as adults we need to be able to interpret aurally, otherwise we can't listen to the radio or use the phone.

Finally, nursery rhymes will help toddlers to draw conclusions from both visual and auditory clues. And research has shown that nursery rhymes are necessary for developing reading skills, so the benefits to introducing all children to rhymes are extensive.

Books

Books are an excellent means of developing communication skills and can be used in many different ways. Here are a few ideas for parents:

1 The best books for developing non-verbal skills in children are those with photos of real people doing real things.

2 Animals and drawings do not have the complexity of facial expressions that humans have and therefore are acceptable but should not be used predominantly.

3 One of the big problems is the paucity of books that use real photos; Margaret Miller's Baby Book series (Miller, 1998) are the best that I have found.

4 Books with mirrors are great for getting the child to copy facial expressions.

5 Sharing information – simply sitting with a book and pointing or talking about different things that can be seen develops early conversational skills of sharing information and showing interest with others. Get the child to point things out too.

6 Talking about what is happening in nursery rhymes or stories through the pictures, and asking questions about what might be about to happen or what people might be talking about, thinking, feeling, and so on, all help to practise theory of mind and other conversational skills.

Games and toys

Games are another very useful tool for developing conversational skills, but only if they are played in a manner that promotes information sharing and enquiry. Children should not just be given things in games because this takes away an opportunity to ask. This is anticipating what is going to happen rather than talking about it and leaving opportunities for the child to join in the conversation. Games are very useful for practising functions of language such as asking for information or answering questions.

If people think about the games they are playing with children as a means of promoting communication, then the child will get the chance to practise her language use.

Imagine playing a posting-type game (there is one for young children called 'Two by Two Game' by Orchard Toys). The goal is to put pairs of animals into the ark. Parents shouldn't just put the cards for posting in pairs on the table in front of the child – all she needs do is pick up the cards that match and post them. No communication need happen at all.

If the parent has the cards nearer them and asks the child, 'Which two animals do you want?', the child will need to ask the adult to pass the cards. This will include naming the animals and using the type of response: 'I want the two elephants' (remember that 'please' should not be insisted on at this stage of communication development). The parents should model the same communication when it is their turn. Get the child to ask the question: 'Which two animals do you want?' and the parent responds: 'I want the two snakes, please'. It is perfectly all right for the parents to model the use of 'please', but they should not demand it from their child.

When posting the cards, encourage the child to say, 'Bye bye horses' or 'Bye bye tigers'. This encourages communication and helps the child to understand that once the cards are posted into the ark they are gone – that is, are finished – see Section 4 for more on beginnings and ends. 'Bye bye' can be used in many situations to promote understanding and communication use.

A game I particularly like – because it promotes non-verbal skills at many different levels – is the 'Guess Who?' game by Hasbro. This is how to play 'Guess Who?' promoting the use of all the non-verbal skills – both interpretation and use. The aim at all times should be for the child to take increasing control of organising the game appropriately – that is, according to how it has been modelled:

- Offer a choice of the coloured boards then give one to each player.

- Shuffle the cards and get the child to pick one.

- Explain the rules of the game.

- Ensure that she knows to keep the identity of her person secret.

- Help her to ask a question such as, 'Is your person a woman?'

- Check that she understands how to answer a yes/no question.

- Make sure the child is looking at the person who is asking a question or responding.

- Answer and confirm with her which people she is going to put down. For instance, say 'No, mine is not a woman' and then help the child to understand that this means that she needs to put down all the women.

- As soon as she has finished putting the women down, get her to look at the person she is playing against so that they know she has finished.

- Make sure she understands that this is the sign that she is ready to be asked a question.

- Then ask the child the next question.

- When she answers, confirm what that means and what will happen as a result. For example, say, 'Yes, yours is a woman' and tell her that you are going to put all the men down.

- Make sure to look at the child when asking the question and also when all the relevant people are put down.

- Looking up when finished is a huge non-verbal sign that it is the child's turn to talk, so this game is a wonderful way of practising the giving and receiving of this sign.

Parents really just need to think differently about games they play with their child and set the game up so that the child needs to ask or give information before making a move. Choosing can be part of the game as well, for example, offering the child a choice of two cards when playing 'Happy Families', and saying 'Which one would you like?' Only give the card when the child asks for it.

Parents should not insist regardless of the circumstances that the child asks for things – at no stage should the child not enjoy what she is doing. If the child has few skills, accept it as a request if she looks at the object or points. As her confidence improves she will start to ask using spoken language.

CONCLUSION

So we have seen how much development is necessary in the area of non-verbal conversational skills throughout this period before the child enters school.

The skills we have looked at are all part of a complex sensibility that she will need to keep developing, even after she has entered school. They include:

- The transfer from early verbal communication skills through to the full use of language, which children should have acquired by about five years.

- The transition from signing to speech.

- Expanding the conversational language function of giving and receiving information.

- Asking for help.

- Being a good listener and speaker.

- Making good sense of increasingly complex facial expressions and body language.

- Understanding all the different emotions as well as the different levels communicated by others.

- Shared knowledge.

- Choice and change.

- Conflict and negotiation.

- Theory of mind.

We have also looked at resources that will help to promote these skills.

If she fails to develop these non-verbal communication skills adequately, then at school she will be very disadvantaged both educationally and socially. She will be less able to function in groups, either small or large ones. In particular, she will find the playground and assembly challenging. But if she develops well in all these areas, then she will have the best prospect of becoming a confident, well-adjusted and able pupil at primary and secondary school.

■ 'LISTEN TO HIM – AND STOP TALKING' ■

PRIMARY DEVELOPMENT 6

Following the rapid and extensive development of non-verbal communication skills in the toddler phase of childhood, entry to school will determine whether the child has sufficient skills to deal confidently with day-to-day events. Only if a child has developed the skills described in the previous two sections will he be able to cope at primary school (KS1, Years 1 and 2)) and have the foundation for further development right through school and well into his teens.

Since the early 1980s in the UK and some other countries, children have been entering school as young as four years of age. This is partly based on the idea that the early acquisition of reading and writing skills will in turn develop their intellectual capacity. In the rest of Europe school entry is usually at six years old, seven in some Scandinavian countries, and these children do no worse and most do even better than children in the UK.

Most children will not have developed sufficient non-verbal skills before they enter school at the age of four – unless their parents have made a big effort to ensure that this has happened – and will have difficulty reaching their potential. Once a child enters school, the drive is often about developing reading and writing skills, to the detriment of non-verbal communication skills.

Many practitioners and research studies recognise that children's communication skills are low on school entry. In my experience, once children are talking well, this concern for their communication disappears. While teachers are aware of the social, emotional and behavioural consequences, they may not attribute them to a communication problem. The pressure to read and write for children with poorly developed non-verbal communication skills can often be too much, with the result that behaviour problems become apparent.

This section will look at what the child should be able to do conversationally at the different stages of primary education and how the transition to junior level requires well-developed conversational skills.

■ PRIMARY SCHOOL

Structure

Teachers are sometimes baffled as to why children take so long to adapt to the changes they encounter on entry to school, particularly as the children to all intents and purposes are able to talk and appear to follow what is going on.

Primary schools try to make it easy for children to make the transition to school, but it is not easy to do if the children have poor communication skills. However, there is more support than teachers might realise for children with poor non-verbal skill development. At school there is more structure and predictability than at home. For those children who are just a little behind in their non-verbal development, this structure and routine may be enough to help them develop the rest of the non-verbal conversational skills they will need over the next few years before junior school entry.

Also, since the associated difficulties have become worse over the past 10–15 years, teachers have adopted many more visual prompts to help the children settle. But before the 1980s, teachers would have expected that within a week or two all the children would have picked up the signals telling them what the teacher wanted and didn't want. The lack of development caused by the social changes described in the opening section make transition a more challenging process for all concerned.

Entry to class – first term

On the first day of term everyone will be a little nervous. But when the teacher explains the timetable – when lunch is and what breaks are all about – this nervousness should start to wane as the child becomes able to predict what will happen. His parents are also likely to have talked through the first day to help his confidence and will have emphasised the fact that at the end of the day he will be met and taken home.

Now all this sounds fine, but unpack it slightly and you will see that the whole day depends on one particular skill – prediction – and this skill depends on the ability to process available non-verbal information.

The child needs to know that the teacher is talking to the whole group, and that it includes him. He will have to remember the information she gives if there is no visual representation of it. He also needs to understand that the other children are as confused as him on this first day. He needs to believe that the teacher is giving useful information. As long as he is able to listen and comprehend what the teacher tells him, then his life will be much easier.

He will also need to know that, because his parents have sent him to school, life at school is not going to be detrimental to him. There should be some non-verbal, subconscious rule that has developed over the previous four or five years that his parents are not going to put him into harmful situations.

Finally, he will need to process all the small non-verbal signals that tell him when an activity ends and another starts, including the body language of teacher and peers, to help him anticipate change.

So although there are many other possible variants, an apparently straightforward situation presents a number of challenges and the child will need to have mastered a range of non-verbal skills in order to survive this first day, let alone the first term.

Structure through signals

The most important factor in helping children in the primary school system is the use of the timetable to tell the child what is going to happen – not only for the next hour or so but until he leaves school at the end of the day. Teachers should not underestimate the benefit of timetables throughout primary education.

They should be clear, visual and accurate. A child with really poor non-verbal understanding needs a timetable visible on his desk. He is unlikely to associate what is written on the board with what he should be doing.

There are other visual and auditory clues that some teachers are increasingly starting to use again following their decline in the 1980s. The daily repetition of the register is one of them. Repetition of anything encourages understanding and structure gives shape to the child's day. However, this is more difficult than you might think. Here is a story about a lad who failed to understand this until he was in his teens!

Case example

I worked with Patrick, a lad of 13 years of age in a secondary school for moderate learning disabilities (which no longer exists). He was showing severe behaviour problems, particularly around registration where he was very disruptive to the whole class.

When I took him aside and asked him about his understanding of the process of registration and the expectations of the teacher about his behaviour, Patrick had absolutely no idea! So I went through it with him, and together we wrote a step-by-step timetable of the registration process. He only needed to use it on a couple of occasions and almost immediately his behaviour improved in this part of the class routine.

However, because he had not picked up this one small aspect of the daily routine that had been repeated regularly since his entry to school at the age of five, his understanding of many other aspects of behaviour for different situations was also very poor.

Patrick needed to benefit from the Not Just Talking intervention to help his understanding – simply showing him the rule and expectation for this one situation did not improve his behaviour in all situations.

So it is important to deal with the expectations of others – his teacher thought Patrick knew what was going on and that he was choosing not to comply.

The real benefit of timetabling is that it helps to further develop the child's predictive skills. Throughout our lives each experience in which we are able to predict successfully adds to our store of knowledge and therefore makes the next prediction in similar circumstances more likely to be accurate. As in the earlier phases of development, if the child fails to pick up easily the signals that tell him what is going on, or is about to happen, then the teacher needs to make those cues bolder and clearer.

Another aspect of structure that may not initially be seen as such is the use of auditory prompts to tell the children when something is about to happen. The most obvious of these is the bell system used in many schools in the UK to tell children and teachers when it is time to change activity, go to break or have lunch, and at the end of the school day. Teachers should draw attention to this use of the bell and what it indicates until certain that all the children in the class fully understand.

Another auditory clue is the clapping of hands. If introduced early and clearly so that the children know exactly what it means, it can be used very successfully. Teachers should not confuse the children by changing the meaning of an auditory clue. For instance, if clapping is established to mean 'Stop and look at me', then it should not be used to mean 'Behave yourself!', for instance.

Later, when the children are very competent at the use of auditory signals, it is possible to vary the meaning of one sound, but I would suggest that some other clue accompanies the sound to indicate a different meaning, such as clapping for wanting the child to stop behaving in a manner inappropriate in the classroom, combined with a follow-up pointing at the child or something similar.

Structure through cloakrooms

Something that teachers may not have thought about as being a visual structure signal is having named pegs in the cloakroom. This is an indication of the child's arrival at school because usually he will have a coat and a bag so there is generally something to put on the peg.

Those working in nursery education have become much more aware of the benefits of this approach, and other clues and markers are commonly used to indicate that the child has arrived or left, such as having the child put a clothes peg with his name on on a line, or hooking a ring on the back of a door when he arrives, then taking it off and putting it in a 'finished' basket when he goes home.

This just increases the number of visual clues signalling the arrival at and departure from school, making it more likely that the child will recognise other more subtle clues associated with these events. Over time the child will pick up these less obvious clues and will no longer require the more marked visual prompts.

At primary school it is likely to be assumed that this level of support is no longer required as the children are that much older. But these aids should not be withdrawn until it is really certain that the child understands fully the routine of arriving at and leaving school.

Because the child usually goes to the toilet on his own or with his peers, this is a difficult area throughout school life. Children who struggle with conversational skill development are vulnerable in situations where there is banter and innuendo. The latter may be less problematic at KS1, but, in the early stages of school entry, a child suddenly has to get used to communal toilets and also cope with the conversations held there – a big difference from home life.

The noise is another factor – this can be amplified in tiled areas. Children with poor non-verbal communication are a bit like non-directional microphones on video cameras. They do not discriminate between helpful and unhelpful noise and so get overloaded with sound. It is inadvisable to leave young children without adult support to survive in any area where peer conversations may cause them undue stress.

Structure through the classroom

Another key part of the structure of the classroom is how the room is organised. The desks are arranged in a certain way and the drawers and cupboards usually have a label on the outside stating what is inside. There are sectioned-off areas in Reception and KS1 classes in the UK. These could be for art, craft, play or construction, but they tend to be dedicated to the subject. The definition of areas into their function communicates clearly what the child is expected to do in that area.

This is another major difference between home and school. Home is much less structured and without a timetable of what is going to happen each day. Activities often happen spontaneously and are unpredictable, such as 'Let's go and see grandad'. Also at home there are not separate areas clearly defined for each activity. Painting, colouring or constructing things may be done at the kitchen table or in the bedroom, for example. Then they are cleared away so that the family can have their lunch or the child can go to bed.

At school the painting area is likely to have paint pots and brushes on the shelf so that when the children look in that direction they quickly learn to understand that painting happens in that area, but this is not the case in the area where reading and writing take place. Because there is less definition at home there is not that clarity, so parents should be encouraged to give other clear signals for the change of activity. Putting on aprons is another clear signal that something messy is going to occur. At this point, parents need to remember to use the 'Time for painting' strategy.

Teachers' expectations

Every teacher will have expectations, either self-imposed or imposed by the National Curriculum, that a child will learn certain things. The child with inadequate non-verbal communication development will struggle to recognise or achieve those expectations.

A real problem may develop as soon as the teacher thinks that the child's behaviour is a result of a deliberate choice to behave in inappropriate ways. Teachers should not come to this conclusion before testing whether or not the child can process non-verbal information in a manner that would mean that he saw things in the same way as his teacher. Only then can anyone be sure that the child is choosing to do what he is doing.

Teachers should not assume that any primary child is shy or doesn't like looking at faces. All children must look at faces for a much longer time than in the past, for all the reasons explained in this book. The teacher must be sure that the child can interpret different emotions and body language before assuming that he just doesn't like looking at people. They should also remember that being able to understand emotions is a precursor skill to being able to communicate about emotions.

Communication issues

All the necessary non-verbal communication developments at this stage of the child's life occur both at home and at school, but because the child spends the majority of his time at school it represents a vital learning ground for good communication development.

Experiential learning

We have already seen the child's need to learn from each situation he enters. This information, which must include who it is he is talking to, where he is and what is going on, is then used to judge how to behave and what to say. Throughout his life at primary school, a child must acquire and store experiential information. The more situations of which he has positive experiences, the more knowledge he accumulates in his subconscious to make good sense of new situations and to respond accordingly. All of this will stand him in good stead when he faces the challenging transition to secondary school.

Speaker and listener

The child will need to improve his skills as both a speaker and a listener in all situations. Until now he has depended on adult support for his communication. Now he must work towards becoming a confident independent speaker and listener, able to give and receive relevant information in whatever situation he finds himself. He should no longer struggle to give appropriate information or responses, no matter who he is talking to.

The skills associated with recognising situational clues will improve for the rest of his life as he accumulates more and more experiential knowledge of conversational situations. As long as he is participating in and attentive to these conversations he will be learning. Any child unable to do this is at risk and should be investigated to establish the extent of his interpretational ability.

Body language

The biggest area of non-verbal communication development at this stage of the child's life is in his understanding and use of complex body language. This can convey the more subtle emotions, such as envy, resentment, concern, and so on, as well as body language that conflicts with what the face communicates, as found in the use of sarcasm.

In sarcasm the verbal message is out of sync with the facial expression and sometimes the body can be communicating something different as well. To the child with limited non-verbal understanding this is confusing and therefore futile.

Styles of conversation

Also developing at this time is the range of styles that a child needs to use for talking to different people, such as the head teacher, class teachers, dinner staff, peers, visitors and the like. Naturally, the child needs to observe how others communicate in these different circumstances for him to be able to use different styles appropriately. This is why it is so important for staff in every department of the school to know that they are models for the children. What they do will be picked up and used in different situations the child encounters, so if the adult uses sarcasm or innuendo, the child may have a bad experience and not learn how to use conversation effectively.

Does he know the message is for him?

A big part of listener skills is knowing that the message includes you when it is given to a group. In class it is sometimes assumed that, if a teacher gives a message to a group of children on the mat or at their desks, everyone knows that the message applies to all the children and not necessarily to the adults in the room. This is a 'rule' that the child should have learned before he entered school, but teachers should not assume he has done so or that he has the skills to process the information she is giving them.

Self - and others awareness

If a child has failed to develop the understanding that other people have different information in their heads from what he has, he will talk to people as though that person has seen exactly the same things as him. For instance, he might say 'Johnny doesn't like her. Will he get into trouble?' He assumes that you both know who Johnny is and what he has done to the girl. This is very noticeable when a child does it all the time and could be very frustrating for his peers. The understanding of self versus others helps us to give the right information in terms of quantity and quality. He may also not realise that other people feel differently from him, so might be surprised when other children cry when he hits them.

Is he able to choose?

It is so easy to think that a child is choosing because he says 'yes' or 'no' in response to a choice. However, it is important to check that he is making an informed choice, which can be done in the following way:

1   Offer a choice between one real option and a bizarre option, for example, 'Would you like to colour or go and eat a bridge?'

2   Offer a choice of two opposites, for example, 'Would you like to colour or wash the floor?'

3   Then if he is able to choose from a positive and negative choice, start to introduce choices where the actions or objects are slightly closer together, for example, 'Would you like to colour or have a drink?' followed by 'Would you like to colour or read a book?' then 'Would you like to colour or play with play-doh ?'

If he is able to choose effectively on a number of occasions between two items that are close together in terms of, say, their function or shape, and then can repeat this on a number of occasions, you will be able to say that he is using choice in an informed way. If not, you will have to make sure that he can do so through elongating any part of this programme.

Groups

Friendships/peer relationships

As we have already seen, conversational skills are central to making and keeping friends. At school it becomes imperative that a child is able to make friends and socialise with his peers. However, holding a conversation with a peer is often the most difficult communication situation for the child. This is due to the fact that talking to adults is much easier as they tend to be accommodating of odd topics and idiosyncrasies displayed by children. They also have greater experience so they can make sense of what a child says more easily, and don't put too many demands on him for specific information if they sense that the child is struggling.

The child's peers, on the other hand, won't pick up the signs of his difficulties. They often find children with poor conversational development too hard to communicate with, and tend to leave these children out of games, or avoid talking to them at all. Children with poor non-verbal communication are snubbed because they:

- talk about what they want to

- are not interested in what others say

- don't listen to what is said to them

- can't answer questions

- can't share information

- don't look at people

- can't keep still.

Another reason for their isolation is that they don't readily perceive social rules or adopt the rules of games easily. This can lead to their being ostracised.

However, children soon learn that those who don't have a good understanding of social situations or who lack confidence in communicating can be useful in certain circumstances. Because they do not recognise when things are about to go wrong, children with non-verbal understanding problems are sometimes left to carry the can.

In these circumstances, in my experience, other more communicatively competent children may talk them into more trouble. Because they are not competent in giving information, the poor communicators may vary their story which may, in any case, have a fundamentally different interpretation from that of their more able peers. So these children are punished more readily and are generally the ones excluded from school if things go really badly.

Non-verbal skills teach us how to behave, resolve problems and deal with conflict. Without full development of these skills, children will have neither the experience nor the skill to negotiate their way out of trouble. Because they are unable to make real friendships, their 'friends' desert them in their hour of need. Later in life this lack of friends can lead to their being vulnerable to exclusion because no one sticks up for them. Also, those doing the excluding often see the child as having chosen to do what he has done and he is blamed as a result.

Groups in the classroom

The definition of a group for school purposes is any situation where there are more than two people present. Children with poor non-verbal communication development find talking to more than one person at a time far too difficult. This is why they often appear to choose to behave badly in such situations. In a one-to-one setting with few distractions, their communication can be quite good.

It is of no use whatsoever to put a child into a class and hope that these skills will rub off on him from interaction with the other children. This is rather like throwing a child into the deep end of a swimming pool with clothes and boots on, and saying, 'Go on, swim!' Without the earlier conversational skills, the child simply won't have the ability to pick up new skills from this complex situation.

This is why children on the autistic spectrum fare much better in class when they sit at a desk facing the wall with side panels to cut out the other children from the child's field of vision. Non-verbal processing is less complex when only one other person is involved, and increases exponentially with the addition of other people. The idea that a child with special needs should be able to cope in a small group is unrealistic if the child has poor non-verbal processing.

At school many children nowadays find talking to more than one person very hard indeed. If they had developed this skill at the appropriate age, they wouldn't find it baffling that on entry to school they can talk to the teacher, but can't talk to their friends in the same effective manner.

Suddenly, in groups, the child has to process non-verbal information from many more people and also pick up more diverse and subtler clues about who is going to speak next and what they are talking about. Therefore the child will probably prefer talking individually to adults who are likely to be more sensitive to their difficulty than children and who usually put less pressure on a child to communicate.

Case example

I have seen quite a few children who do not cause any problems at all at home and whose parents find it hard to understand when there are problems with behaviour at school.

This is usually for two reasons, the most common being that the child is a singleton. Therefore there is no competition for his parents' attention from siblings and the parents' life is usually dedicated to this one child.

The other reason is similar but occurs less often – I have only come across this on a couple of occasions. Amir's parents had realised from an early stage that interacting with their child caused problems, and decided that the best tactic was to leave him to his own devices. So when he came home from school he would go straight up to his room and play on the computer, watch TV or do something else that didn't involve talking to anyone. Amir would only come down to eat and went straight back upstairs afterwards.

If there were any family activities the parents would put absolutely no pressure on him to conform – basically he was allowed to do what he wanted. Without pressure the child has no need to resort to the behaviours that he has developed to get himself out of conversations he is unable to understand.

At school, he would not be allowed to choose to do something different as children are there to follow the curriculum. So this pressure to conform would cause a reduction in his ability to behave appropriately.

The number of people being spoken to has a direct impact on the complexity of the interpretation and therefore children with poor interpretational skills will find understanding and talking in groups much more difficult. Communicating in groups of two or three people is generally easier than larger groups, such as at playtime (see below) or assembly, which can be particularly challenging. It is easy for teachers to assume that if a child can function adequately in a small group of no more than three, he can therefore cope in larger groups. This is rarely the case. Larger groups require much more complex processing of non-verbal information than groups of three because you have to look at and interpret the information from more and disparate sources. Also, a combination of peers and adults will make a difference.

School assembly is an area of significant challenge in terms of non-verbal understanding because of the unspoken rules and expectations involved in the process. The child, who has probably never experienced activities in a spacious room with a large number of children and a few adults, will have to develop more sophisticated skills to cope with this situation. Breaking down the component non-verbal 'rules' for a school assembly shows the complexity of this activity compared with smaller groups or one-to-one conversations. In order to function well getting to and from assembly, as well as during it, the child will need to:

1   understand what time of the day or week assembly usually takes place

2   understand the instruction to get ready to go to assembly

3   know what the queue is for; how to take his place in the queue; how to behave in a queue

4   understand the direction the queue is pointing in so he knows whether it is going into or out of the classroom – many children who require Not Just Talking's intervention don't know how to 'read' direction

5   know that he should follow the class teacher (in the queue) to the hall

6   notice the class teacher's non-verbal clues of showing the class to sit and where to do so

7   predict what else might happen

8   predict what the speaker might talk about

9   look at the speaker

10 ignore everyone else but maybe keep the class teacher in peripheral vision

11 know how to address the head teacher, rather than a class teacher who he knows much better

12   recognise the need to keep quiet and sit still

13 notice signals to get up at the end of assembly/when it is time to sing/time to clap, etc

14 use queuing rules again to get back to class

15 predict what will happen back at class – what is expected.

I have not covered in detail all the situations where non-verbal understanding would tell you how to behave – much will depend on what happens during the event – but the examples given should help you understand the non-verbal demands on the child of just this one activity. Other equally challenging situations happen throughout the child's day; breaking down the components in this way helps to reveal how challenging they can be to children with poorly developed non-verbal skills.

Remember that all situations that challenge the child's ability to understand what is happening, or to predict what will happen next, will cause a change in his communicative behaviour or force him to resort to verbal or physical aggression or other behaviours that he adopts to get himself out of the situation. As we are now going to see, playgrounds are just as complex, but in a slightly different way.

Playground

The playground can be a place where conversational skills develop further. Playing with other children of all ages helps the child to observe many kinds of interaction – telling stories to peers or making up games, talking to helpers, calming an argument down, reporting something to an adult. The playground is often a more difficult arena than, say, assembly because it involves mainly interacting with peers rather than adults.

Watching all these things helps the child to develop his understanding of the conventions associated with different forms of play – and different types of conversation. The child needs to know in which situations to apply 'rules' that are particular to that set of circumstances, ie, rules within rules that depend on, say, a person's presence, a change in the game being played, the time of day, whether it's someone's birthday, and so on.

However, because early opportunities for non-verbal communication skill development have decreased, playgrounds have become a most difficult place for a child. He is unable to learn all the complex rules pertaining to the playground because he hasn't developed the earlier skills that would enable him to do so. This mostly relates to the simple fact that children do not look at people sufficiently today.

One effect of not looking at people is that children do not learn how to resolve conflicts – so they don't learn what works and what doesn't work and as a result don't benefit from trying out negotiation. I have even known children who have never witnessed an argument at home. If parents don't teach their children how to resolve differences at home, it is not surprising that they are unable to do so when they reach school.

When you get a large group of children playing together but not necessarily the same game, the level of complication increases. The child will have to identify and interpret many more variations in body language. On top of this, children may have to deal with the poor or limited use of body language and other associated communication problems of other children in their peer group.

Conflict often arises because a child fails to pick up the visual or aural signs that a game has finished or that the game is no longer fun. So again we see how fundamental is the skill of identifying, interpreting and processing the non-verbal information in situations.

A child will only find himself able to cope in a negotiation situation when he has developed good understanding of these complex situations. The next challenge is that the ability to negotiate is a very high-level conversational skill which children going into school are only just learning about.

Differences between home and school

At home, parents should have demonstrated through communicative experiences with their child that there are different ways of talking to people. This should include getting angry and how to resolve arguments effectively through negotiation. Without this experience at home, children will not be able to apply the knowledge in school interactions either in the class or in the playground.

Teachers should only think that the child is choosing to talk and behave appropriately if they are certain that the child has sufficient non-verbal communication skills. A child who behaves very differently in another situation will not possess good interpretational skills. Teachers should check that the child knows how to communicate and behave appropriately in all situations.

Teachers should also be aware that, if a parent is saying that the child behaves differently at home and is disrupting family life, they are telling the truth even if the child is perfectly behaved at school. As we have seen, the structure at school may be sufficient for the child to 'survive' during the school day. It is not the parents' fault as at the time of writing (June 2011) there are no books telling them how to develop these non-verbal skills.

Consistency

In the past it didn't really matter if dinner staff or teachers in the playground remonstrated with the children in a different manner. Children had the ability to adjust quickly and soon would know the differences and similarities of non-verbal communication between different people. However, some children now enter school with such poor communication that there is a greater need for consistency of approach from school staff. All staff should use the same form or words and style to praise or admonish children. All the different styles of communication used throughout the day should also be very clear and simple for children to pick up. This will help them to try out the styles and hopefully use them appropriately. Adults should particularly avoid the use of sarcasm.

Consistency of approach is also very necessary. A child who is trying out a new communication skill will not progress if there is only one person in the school who recognises the skill. During Not Just Talking's intervention it is recommended that children ask for help in the playground rather than take the situation into their own hands. If those on duty do not understand that this is the approach to be adopted, their reaction might be the opposite of what is required. This will confuse the child and signal to him that the communicative strategy he has been given is less useful than the behaviour of hitting out at his peers – which the new communication method was intended to replace. It is our role as good communicators to facilitate the child's communication and 'sell' him the concept that communication is a more efficient method of achieving what he wants than, for instance, hitting out at others.

So consistency of approach is vital to help children develop new skills, and all staff at school should be modelling behaviour that they wish the child to adopt.

Academic pressure

There is a direct relationship between the child's ability to communicate in all situations and his ability to learn at school. Most lessons are delivered through conversations – any situation where a message is being given to a person or group of people is a conversation. So children with poor non-verbal understanding will not be able to participate effectively in learning and therefore won't achieve their potential. As a result they will experience more pressure, which in turn will cause these children to withdraw or become disruptive.

As we will see in the next section, increasing academic demands may reduce a child's ability to make good sense of situations. As a result his behaviour may deteriorate and he might opt out of talking or taking part in the activity. So once again, development in another skill area – apparently unrelated – is dependent on the child first developing his non-verbal conversational skills.

Developments outside school

At home, parents should make sure that their child doesn't spend all his time looking at screens. At this age a child needs to experience many activities with many different sets of peers so that he can build on and extend the skills that he should be developing in the playground. Of course, if he hasn't developed these skills at an earlier stage, he won't be able to do this without the intervention.

Mixed-ability classes: strategies to use in class

In order to be able to deal with a mixed-ability class, children need good conversational skill development.

A summary of what works and what doesn't:

1   Be clear and specific in what you say, leaving no possibility that the child might

misinterpret the message, so 'Eat now', not 'Would you like to eat your cabbage now please?' This last message may not only confuse the child but leaves an option for the child to answer 'No!', thus setting up a situation of conflict that he won't be able to deal with appropriately.

2   When the child is no longer confused by verbal messages it is possible to revert to more usual requests. But you may find that being clear and specific is so effective that you stick with the clarity of message giving advised here.

3   Use bold and obvious visual or auditory clues at every opportunity. Draw the child's attention to them. Make sure he knows what they mean and what they signal.

4   Keep these signals consistent, always conveying the same thing.

5   Do not use innuendo, idioms or sarcasm. To be able to understand such messages, the child will need to be able to 'read' the hidden meaning behind the words. Without this skill they will be terribly confused and are likely to interpret the words literally, for instance, 'Put a sock in it!' When his non-verbal skills improve he will be better able to understand hidden meanings.

6   Repeat the same clear message until the child complies, for example, 'I want you to sit still'; 'I want you to sit still'. (The use of the phrase 'I want you to' is effective because, when used consistently, the child will not even need to listen to it and will just focus on the last word or two to get the meaning.) Don't be tempted to change the message, to 'Will you please sit still' or 'Sit where you are told', etc.

7   When a child does something positive, ensure that whoever is praising him tells him which behaviour he is being praised for. Generic words such as 'Well done', 'Brilliant' or 'That was really good' are not specific enough for children with poor non-verbal understanding. They need their attention drawn directly to the good behaviour so that they are more likely to repeat it in a similar situation. Instead, say 'Good eating' or 'Good waiting', for example. It is possible to add words such as 'That was good eating' or 'Good waiting, John'. However don't make the phrases any longer than this or the message will be complicated and the child less likely to understand.

8   With regard to the use of 'please', do not insist on this until the child's non-verbal communication skills have reached a four- or five-year-old level.

9   Always ensure that children are looking at you before giving them important information.

10 Don't accept 'yes' as an answer from a child with social, emotional and behaviour problems. Check out with the child that he has understood what you want him to do by asking him to tell you what he is going to do. This helps prevent confrontation when things don't go quite as you expect. It will also give you an insight into how confusing the child finds the world.

11 When something does go wrong, for example, they stand too close to people when talking to them, remember that, if the child is simply told to stop the behaviour, he

may not have an understanding of what it is appropriate to do in that situation. Always tell them what it is you want them to do, for instance, 'I don't want you to stand so close when I am talking to someone else. I want you to stand this far away' and demonstrate how far by either standing there yourself or making the gap obvious with your hands. This technique can be used in all sorts of situations, such as hitting other children, throwing objects, talking out of turn, etc.

12 When the child shows any sign of inappropriate verbal or social behaviour, it indicates that his confusion has reached a state where he can no longer cope. Being given too much spoken information has confused him and therefore talking to him at this stage will make the situation much worse – more words simply adding to his confusion and frustration. If the early signs of confusion are recognised, this technique is easy to use. Sometimes the child might be very clear and, when first becoming confused, say something like 'Don't talk to me!' Please listen to him and stop talking to him. Even if the child is in a very distressed state, just say calmly and reassuringly to him 'When you are ready to talk, we will talk'. Then leave him on his own. No one else should interact with him either. Don't go too far away – it is imperative that the child is kept safe at this time. Initially ask 'Are you ready to talk?' quite regularly – every 10–20 seconds. People who know the child will be able to judge the level of repetition necessary. Some children need asking every minute or two or longer. If he says 'no', he must be left alone. Even if he doesn't say 'no' but indicates in some other way, perhaps by pushing the person away or shouting obscenities, take this as a 'No'! He alone can get himself out of his state of confusion. If this strategy is used consistently, very soon he will say almost immediately 'I'm ready' when told 'When you are ready to talk, we will talk' and get back to whatever he had been doing. Then it is possible to talk to him. If the child is very confused and anxious, do not talk about the situation that has sent him into the confused state, nor talk about what he might do better next time. Only talk through the cause of his behaviour if you are certain he is calm enough and will understand. Otherwise change the topic to something you know the child will be confident and happy to talk about.

13 Don't attempt to sweeten what is being communicated through the use of sarcasm or 'politeness'.

14 Don't insist on the use of 'sorry' until the child's non-verbal understanding improves significantly. Otherwise he will just learn to respond parrot-fashion and have no real understanding of why he is apologising. In time, once intervention has started, he will automatically start to use 'sorry' appropriately. Here is a story about what happens if 'sorry' is insisted on.

Case example

David's parents were insistent that their son said sorry when he came back downstairs after an outburst.

Eventually, he would just come downstairs and say sorry, but still had outbreaks of bad

temper which puzzled the parents. This was because David had not learned the meaning of sorry or what it related to. So he continued to do what it was his parents didn't want him to do.

Because they thought that he knew what sorry meant David was set up to fail as in fact he had no idea what it meant – he was just saying the word without meaning.

Strategies that won't work

Any strategy either based on behaviourist techniques or designed to promote the child's verbal understanding or expression will fail because the child will be unable to generalise what he is being told in one situation and apply it appropriately to another. Behaviourist techniques are based on the principle that communication and behaviour are learned through a stimulus–response process. A child is stimulated by something he sees and then responds in some way.

This approach doesn't work with a child with poor non-verbal skills because he is unable to recognise the signals telling him what it is that defines appropriate behaviour for that particular situation. The following case history illustrates this point.

Case example

Jason had been excluded from mainstream school at an early age and his parents had put him into private education in the belief that smaller classes would suit him better. This is often the reaction of parents and, as these parents found out, it rarely resolves the problem – this lad was on the verge of exclusion from his fee-paying school.

The reason why such children are excluded from private schools is twofold:

1   As we have already seen, groups of any size are problematic for children with non-verbal processing difficulties. Although the class size of this school was smaller, the day-to-day routine was the same as a state primary school, ie, he had to join in group activities.

2   The parents of other children who are paying large sums for the education of their children tend to be quite vociferous with regard to those who are disrupting their children's attention and reducing their ability to get on with their work. Pressure is put on the senior management who see the potential loss of pupils in financial terms. For them it is preferable to remove one child than lose four or five or more.

Both these reasons applied in the case of Jason. On assessment his interpretation of emotions was extremely poor and he had no idea how to weigh up possible responses in his mind and choose a behaviour appropriate to the circumstances.

On my arrival at the school, I was very impressed at the level of visual structure employed. Jason was walking round the school with a timetable in his pocket of every lesson during the week. At the end of each lesson he had to give the timetable to the teacher (because it was a fee-paying school, there was an added complication in KS2 in that he had more than one teacher per day). The teacher would then give him a down, sideways or up arrow for his behaviour during the lesson.

For a couple of sessions, I asked him how the card was going and he looked despondent and said 'All down arrows'. The following session he came in smiling from ear to ear and spontaneously told me that he had got an up arrow! I then asked what he had got the up arrow for. His face changed and he said 'I don't know'.

It is easy to see that the school had unwittingly set Jason up to fail:

1 *The teacher who gave him the up arrow thinks the child knows which behaviour it applied to.*

2 *The child can't make out, in a lesson of 45 minutes to an hour, which particular behaviour the teacher liked. There may well have been some behaviours during the lesson that the teacher didn't like at all. The child with poor conversational skills does know that he can ask the teacher to clarify this for him.*

3 *The teacher may even have told him which behaviour he was getting the arrow for, but in the movement from this lesson to the next and over the course of the weekend, the child had no memory of what the teacher had said. This is partly due to the transitory nature of speech and the child only having an arrow to remind him how to behave.*

4 *However, even if he had remembered which behaviour she liked, he then would have to recognise the signals telling him when it was appropriate to use that behaviour again. If he were to choose to use it again inappropriately his teacher would not be pleased and he would be back to square one.*

5 *The teacher may have gone back to the staffroom and said 'At last Jason has behaved well during my lesson.' The teacher also may have shared this information about the behaviour with all the other teachers, so setting the child up for failure in every other lesson because their expectations would have been lifted. They would anticipate better behaviour. But he would still be unable to replicate the behaviour because he didn't understand what he had done to please the first teacher.*

6 *The tiny grain of confidence that he had gained is now dispelled and the likelihood of his being excluded has increased.*

Just telling him what he had done well, but also giving him visual feedback for the behaviour the teacher wanted him to repeat that he could carry round, telling him exactly what the good behaviour was, would increase the likelihood of Jason being able to repeat the behaviour in another lesson.

So here you have all the strategies to use and those to avoid. In my experience, using unsuccessful strategies leads to a highly stressed, frustrated and deskilled workforce in schools – they are doing what they have been told, but despite their best efforts nothing appears to work with these children. Once these strategies are implemented consistently, teachers will be amazed at the change.

Transfer to a new class

The expectation of most teachers now is that there will be a period of at least a term where children are 'settling in' to the new routine. Some children will take longer. This is not normal development. Children with good non-verbal interpretation skills should only need a week or two at the most to adjust to the new teacher and classroom.

We have seen in the early sections of normal development how important skills of prediction and understanding change are and how these are based on the sound development of non-verbal interpretation.

The child's smooth transition between classes is dependent on knowing what is going to happen in the next class/year – amongst other skills he will need the ability to predict accurately and with confidence. He will only make a successful transition if he understands most of the implications of the move and is able to quickly familiarise himself with and read the mannerisms and body language of the next teacher.

■ KEY STAGE 2/JUNIOR

The next three years of primary education are mostly focused on preparing for secondary education. Expectations of academic capability and behaviour increase. This adds to the pressure on the child and, if his non-verbal skills are not well developed, he will struggle. This struggle will lead to his adopting a range of tactics for getting himself out of situations and out of trouble. If his prediction skills were really good by this age, they would help him to know how to avoid confrontation.

All the skills from this point rely on earlier learning and experience so if the child hasn't developed those skills, he will not achieve his potential.

Transition to Key Stage 2

Any child will find this transition a bit of a challenge to his communication skills. However, with good development, as already stated, this should not be a problem. In a child who is able to talk, any sign of difficulty can be a warning signal that his non-verbal skills might be underdeveloped.

So teachers just need to be aware of the difficulties that will be posed when new and more complex concepts are introduced. Do not assume that children are keeping up with the additional information load. Good teachers always check out the children's understanding. There are different ways of doing this:

- The teacher asks a child she knows to be struggling to explain what he is going to do. For example, if the request has been for the children to put their books away and go and get their gym bags to change for gym, he should be able to tell her all this information.

- The teacher gets the children to work in groups of two or three to tell each other what is going to happen.

- A child from one group is asked to go and tell the children in another group what they need to do.

- Listeners can evaluate whether the message is the same as the one they heard.

This can be done at any stage of the child's development as long as no assumptions are made about the child's ability to understand what is being asked of him. Remember to use all the strategies outlined in this section. It is better to go back to basics rather than talk at a level beyond the child's skill.

CONCLUSION

In this section we have covered all the non-verbal skills that a child will need to possess to ensure that he can cope with entry to primary school, move from class to class, move up to KS2 and be ready for the greater challenge posed to his non-verbal communication skills by entry to secondary school.

We have seen how children should enter school with sufficient communication skills to enable them to cope with the transition to their first class. We looked at the importance of structure in the classroom and the school routine, and how to enhance that structure to make things easier for children who might not have sufficient skills. We also saw how teacher expectations may not be in sync with what children are actually capable of doing and how these expectations may be driven by the National Curriculum and SATS tests.

I stressed the importance of experiential learning at this stage of a child's life and how it would not be achieved if the child's non-verbal interpretational skills were limited. We looked at how much more the child has to learn at this stage about understanding and using body language.

Talking to more than one person is a far more demanding skill than talking to an adult for children with non-verbal difficulties. Children should not be expected to pick up skills just by being part of a group. Only when their skills in the one-to-one setting are good can they be expected to learn the more complex skills associated with talking in a group.

The complications of assembly and the playground were analysed and the importance of consistency among the whole staff for the purposes of developing different styles of communication in children and also to encourage the use of new skills.

It was pointed out that a lack of structure could make home a far more complex place with regard to non-verbal interpretation and that parents who describe the poor behaviour of a child at home should be listened to, even if the child behaves perfectly at school.

The impact of academic pressure as the child progresses through the school system and the effect on behaviour was discussed. Finally, effective strategies were described and there was explanation of why some common approaches just don't work with children who have failed to developed non-verbal communication skills.

'**TURBULENT TIMES**'

TEENAGE DEVELOPMENT

7

One of the main transitions in a child's life, in which her non-verbal communication skills are tested to the maximum, occurs when she moves from an educational model in which the class is taught by a single teacher to one in which she will have contact with several subject teachers each day.

There are a few exceptions in the UK. In the private sector this change to more than one teacher might happen at KS2 or, in the middle school system, when the transition occurs in Year 5 (nine years of age). Of course, job sharing and supply cover may happen in any school, but the basic difference is between a relationship with one or two teachers in primary school and relationships with a number of teachers for different subjects at secondary school.

The majority of children in the UK make the change in Year 6. They go into the much more complex non-verbal environment in Year 7 when the child is 11 (if that is before 31 August of that year). This section will look at the changes in the child's communication at this time.

What you should be looking for as normal development at this age is signs that the child is picking up all the non-verbal information around her, processing it correctly and storing it effectively for use in comparable situations. She should soon be able to apply the newly learned appropriate behaviours for each lesson or situation. But there are hurdles she will have to negotiate in order to develop sufficient non-verbal processing skills.

SECONDARY SCHOOL

As the majority of children go to state secondary schools, I will use this as the main model for the purposes of this section. However, there will be information about exceptions in separate subsections below.

The model for mainstream secondary schools in the state system comprises:

- large numbers of children compared with primary school

- subject teachers, ie, more than one teacher per day

- large buildings with many classrooms

- circuitous routes between buildings for different lessons

- large playing fields – plenty of outside space in which to get lost or confused and far away from adult support

- higher levels of academic pressure in working toward GCSE-level exams in Years 10 and 11.

Seen from the perspective of a child of perhaps just 11 years of age, this is a massive change all at once. Schools try their hardest to make this change as easy as possible, but most of this support is based on the assumption that the child has good non-verbal communication skills. If told something clearly then she should understand. However, not all – in fact, only a few – children have the skill level necessary to give them a chance to make the transition well.

Take, for example, a situation in which timetabling pressures mean that a maths lesson has to move to an art room. Think of the confusing situational clues in that setting: the teacher is not the one usually associated with the subject taught in that room; the surroundings are not those associated with the maths lesson; the timing is not what the child associates with being in that room or taking that route to class. For a child with non-verbal communication difficulties, this could be extremely unsettling and perplexing.

Transition pressure

When moving to secondary school, a child will sometimes make the transition with friends. But she might not be with anyone she knows; this will depend to some extent on:

- the sheer numbers of children in that intake

- her subject choices

- the child's educational potential.

As a result she may end up in a class of 30 or more children, of whom she may know only one or two.

School life

The school site will be much larger and her lessons may be in completely different parts of the building or campus. So the child may find it a daunting task to find her way quickly and in a timely fashion to the next lesson. For a child facing the challenges posed by secondary education, life will be much easier if she is able to talk through issues related to finding her way round the school. These might include:

- getting to class on time

- having the right books and equipment for the lesson, such as her PE clothes, in her bag

- the best method of talking to teachers and dealing with their expectations

- coping with the homework, and so on.

After the first few lessons, her teachers will expect her to know what to bring with her. It is likely that the teacher told her in the previous lesson what she needed, so failure to bring the correct books or equipment might be interpreted as negligence.

Also, possibly for the first time, she will rub shoulders with much older and larger children wandering round the school corridors. They may seem quite intimidating to her as many of them will be near their full adult height. These teenagers may make comments about the younger and smaller Year 7 intake that she may not understand: she may become anxious or frightened as a result. Being able to communicate effectively will help her because she can voice her feelings to her form teacher, or to her peers who may be experiencing the same sort of disorientation. Listening to what others say will help her to develop her own strategies and rules for these new situations.

Moreover, the older children are not likely be interested in primary school conversations for too long. She quickly needs to learn – from the non-verbal signals – which topics are acceptable and which are not. She needs to learn to read the body language that tells her not to persist with a topic, or to get out of the situation when something might be about to happen that she can't deal with or doesn't want to be part of.

All these factors militate against the child's best efforts to 'fit in'. Her most useful strategy is to make friends with some of the children who share all her lessons, so that they can act as a visual reference and support her in difficult situations around the school. Of course, this ability to make friends also depends on how well developed her non-verbal communication skills are.

Making friends

Throughout the book we have seen how conversational skills are central to being able to make and keep friends: it is on entry to secondary school that these skills must come into their own. A child who has not acquired all the skills she needs will be at a disadvantage.

The mere act of sharing information with others who are experiencing the same sort of pressure will help her begin to develop an understanding and tactics for coping with this new situation. Children at secondary school need to be able to share information about coping – how to find things or how to deal with new or different situations. Sharing helps to make life at school easier and will give whoever is part of the conversation some other approaches to try out. By this stage the child should have the ability to understand which strategies to adopt and which ones she may need to let go because they haven't worked.

Friends will also give warnings of what different teachers expect and how they behave, information that can be invaluable in helping to keep the child in the teachers' good books. Those children who do not benefit from this type of advice or support may quickly find themselves on the wrong side of certain teachers. From that point on, it is hard to put things right unless the child's conversational skills are up to scratch.

 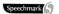

Academic pressure

Another change to do with life at secondary school is that the academic routine and demands are much greater. The child will have to focus on individual subjects rather than learn about them through activities and projects, as in primary school. This focus on subjects requires increasing attention to detail and the need to conform to certain standards of presentation and engagement, all of which add to the pressure on the child to understand and keep up.

As we have seen, pressure and stress are two of the greatest inhibitors of the use of good communication. For more about this see Section 6.

Teachers' expectations

It is very easy for teachers to think that, because a child is able to talk well, she understands everything that is said to her, no matter what the situation. This assumption about the child's understanding can lead to false expectations and to her responses being misconstrued.

The teacher might think that, if the child behaves in an unexpected manner or uses a behaviour for which she has been reprimanded on a previous occasion, she has chosen to behave in that manner. This is an unspoken and therefore hidden assumption by the teacher. As adults we see the visual clues, link them to our past experience and make a judgement about how to act or react. Sometimes we get it wrong. A child with poor non-verbal skills may have difficulty making these connections in the first place.

In my experience, teachers at secondary level tend not to check with the child what made them behave in a particular way. If they did they might be quite surprised! By just asking the child the simple question 'What made you think/do/say that?' they would open up the possibility of a different response from the child which would help the teacher to understand her confusion.

As a teacher you would respond differently to a child you know to be confused by what is going on around her from how you would respond to one you suspect of choosing to be difficult. Because all our behaviour is predicated on how we see the world and how we interpret what we see, a child cannot be deemed to be choosing a behaviour if we do not know which particular signals she was focused on or what understanding she had of the situation.

To help illustrate how easy it is to misunderstand people's actions, look at the following example.

English is a subject that is likely to cause more difficulties for children with non-verbal problems because it is not a 'black-and-white' subject, ie, answers to questions are not simply 'yes' or 'no'. In an English lesson the teacher asks for the children reading Skellig by David Almond to sit quietly and read pages 3–6 and says that she will be asking questions later about what they have read. Those who are reading The Monster Garden by Vivien Alcock are told by the teacher that they should answer the questions on the whiteboard.

Anna missed the instruction completely as she was distracted by something else in the classroom. In any case, she is not really aware of which group she belongs to and therefore which book she should be reading.

She sees most of the other children getting out their books and opening them and then remembers that on another occasion, getting out her book and making comments about the pictures had made the other children laugh – the teacher had been out of the room at that time. So she may think this behaviour would be good to use in this situation. She has not recognised the key difference that the teacher is present this time.

The English teacher is likely to think that Anna is choosing to behave as she does in order to be provocative or disruptive or to attract attention. The teacher may then react in a way that also assumes that the child understands the normal 'rule' of behaviour in this particular situation.

Making assumptions such as these sends us down a route where the child is less and less likely to be able to communicate. The child becomes increasingly confused because what she and the teacher thought was a fairly straightforward situation has turned into a complex challenge.

Generally, the consequence of this is a deterioration in behaviour. The child is admonished for behaving in a particular manner because of a misinterpretation of what is actually going on by both parties. The child's intention is likely not have been to upset the teacher but this is the outcome. Moreover, the child is expected to have the skills to deal with the consequences of an action that she didn't understand in the first place!

When there is a mismatch between the child's actions and the teacher's expectations, there is potential for conflict of one sort or another. Remember that these expectations can be slightly different in each class because of the different teachers involved. This complicates the issue even more for the child. If her conversational skills are compromised then the outcome of the situation is likely to result in a further decline in the child's behaviour, not an improvement.

Benefits of the middle school model

Some local education authorities in the UK have adopted a middle school system. This means that, instead of moving up to secondary school in Year 7, children move to middle school in Year 5. They then stay there until Year 8, ie, 9–13 years of age, before moving to secondary school.

This model has quite a few benefits for the development of non-verbal communication skills. The main one is that children do not have to compete with others who are older than 13 and so have time to consolidate and develop new experiential skills.

Another benefit relates to the number of teachers that the children see. This is reduced to 9–10 in middle schools compared with at least 10 in the secondary school model. This reduction in the number of teachers alone will give the child a better chance of learning the body language of her teachers. Sometimes the teachers may have been known to the child over the previous few years if the middle school is on the same site. This of course is a much better model than throwing the child in at the deep end at secondary school in a new location, with all new teachers and perhaps new peers as well.

Independent school model

This model usually has the change to subject teachers much earlier, at KS2. Although it is similar to the middle school model, the fact that the change takes place at an earlier age could be detrimental to the child's communication development.

A benefit is that in a small school environment:

- the child will know, or know of, the teachers that she has at KS2

- her peers should be the same and the number of children in the class is usually lower than in a state school

- not all lessons will be subject based, so for those lessons she will be mixing with her tutor group, who she has probably known since entry to the school.

However, there are some downsides which will eventually outweigh the positive factors:

- Many children enter independent schools because they have been on the point of exclusion from state schools as a result of their behaviour.

- This set of children will add a mix to the group which may cause a few challenges, but usually they don't stay at the independent school for too long.

- The other factor that makes the independent school model difficult for children with poor non-verbal communication skills is that the academic pressure increases exponentially at KS2. This is because many of these schools are focused on getting children into private secondary schools; they are therefore known as 'preparatory' or 'prep' schools.

As we have already seen, the combination of academic pressure and the need to develop good non-verbal communication skills in order to help cope with this pressure is often too great for the child. The same outcome applies:

- the child's behaviour deteriorates

- teachers try to help

- the child's behaviour gets worse

- teachers can't cope

- there is pressure from other parents

- the child is excluded.

It is a real shame that children who would benefit from just a small amount of intervention should end up being excluded so often from whichever school system they find themselves in.

 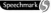

Communication development during adolescence

Some big steps in non-verbal communication skill development are necessary in the period between 11 and 16 years, without which the child may become extremely vulnerable. This period coincides with the huge changes that boys and girls go through in their physical and emotional development as they prepare to enter the adult phase of their life.

Here are some changes that relate particularly to children's ability to enhance their non-verbal communication skills and ideas about what adults need to do to ensure smooth passage through this difficult time.

Emotional change

When a child enters puberty (and this seems to be happening earlier) she is flung into a mass of emotional and physical changes. Unless really good non-verbal understanding is developed at an earlier stage in the child's life, she will find these changes extremely hard to handle. Even children who are proficient communicators find this period of life difficult and confusing. She will need to make particular strides in understanding:

- relationships between people

- what people might be thinking

- different levels of emotions

- new emotional experiences

- other people's changing perceptions of her.

The challenges of puberty are greatest in relation to emotional development. In my opinion, it is this confused emotional state that causes the child to sink into depression.

In normal development the child will need to recognise and adjust to the surging emotions that suddenly start to appear: if she hasn't been able to learn about other more basic emotions, these strong feelings and urges may shock and confuse her. She will then need to be able to name the emotion and recognise it in others, particularly her peers. Finally, she will need to know how to deal with the feeling appropriately. By talking through these changes with her friends and family she will gradually be able to come to terms with her turbulent feelings.

Not only will she need to understand powerful and different emotions but she will also need to cope with the changing nature of her relationships with peers, children of the opposite sex and members of her family. As the child matures into a young person, her role in the family will change and, particularly for girls, the reaction of her parents will communicate to her their concerns about her happiness, safety and sexuality. With good non-verbal interpretation she will be better equipped to handle these changes satisfactorily.

Physical change

The child's body changes a great deal at this time too, so her self-image will alter and she will need to become comfortable in her 'new' body. This self-image is so important because it helps to build self-esteem. This in turn leads to confidence and composure – an essential component of good communication.

In boys the changes include a specific change to body image which is different from girls' – the alteration of the larynx. The growth spurt at this time affects the length of the boy's vocal cords and as consequence there is a change in the sound of his voice. This deepening of his voice brings with it a complete change to his self-image, underlining his masculinity. He has to cope with the variation in pitch while this transition happens and then adapt to his new 'manly' voice when it settles at the target pitch.

Although these changes do not in themselves directly impact on the development of non-verbal skills, they do have a part to play in the total development of the child, so will impact on communication. As long as the child is confident and happy, she will continue to accumulate the skills that she needs to help her communicate whatever the situation.

Social impact

Becoming a young woman (or a young man) will affect all teenagers' relationships – with other girls and boys, with family, with adults. The process of growing into adults begins in their early teens but carries on until the end of their teens and in boys continues for a while into their twenties. This is a long period of time and all the while they will be adjusting their relationships and behaviour according to what they are able to learn from their experiences – much of which, as we have seen, is gained by absorbing non-verbal information.

But this happens only if their non-verbal skills are developing 'normally'. Any lack of skill at this stage will have a big effect on their life chances.

Family relationships

For a girl the main difference will be that she becomes much more interested in making herself attractive to boys and all that this entails. Her relationship with her father will change too, as the more sexually attractive she becomes, the more his role is to help her to learn the social rules about contact with the opposite sex.

So as a younger girl it might have been perfectly normal for him to help wash and dress her, but after her body starts to change this will have ceased and her father will demonstrate this change by not rushing into her room but knocking to make sure that she is in a suitable state of dress. This is not 'prissy' or to be looked on as in any sense regressive, but is an important step in his daughter learning how to present her 'new' body in a manner that is appropriate to the person she is with and the situation – not always an easy development and one which may take many years to get right. But if the parents aren't aware of their role in developing their child's understanding at this time then she might get the wrong messages entirely.

The challenges to the family at this time, as the child becomes increasingly independent of her parents, require her non-verbal understanding to be sufficiently developed to appreciate that, although her parents are arguing with her about what time she needs to come home at night, they still love her. At different times they will talk to her in styles other than chiding or shouting.

Peer relationships

These relationships will also change as children grow and boys and girls may start to be interested in very different things, such as football, make-up, video games or pop stars. Boys and girls may grow apart at this stage, but when they come back together at about 14 years, they will all have changed – they will be interested in new things and may start looking at each other in new ways. The child's non-verbal understanding needs to be well developed to cope with this change in peer relationships.

Developing a sexual understanding

This is one of the most complex areas of development that a child will go through and if her non-verbal skills are in any way underdeveloped she will not manage the transition well.

A child needs to learn quickly the particularly subtle cues that body language and facial expression reveal to let her know whether someone else:

- finds her attractive

- is showing sexual interest

- is uninterested

- is interested in another person.

She will need to understand that all this is going on around her and quickly learn what signals she can and can't make. For boys, this is often a more bewildering art and as they grow it will become more important that they correctly read and interpret the clues given out by girls. Remember that boys find identifying and correctly interpreting these signals harder than girls and the consequences of not doing so can be serious.

Teacher relationships

The complications of relationships, mainly between teenage girls and male teachers, is also thrown into the mix during this phase of development. This is all to do with the developing sexuality of young people and their lack of experience in how to communicate or react to it.

Attractive young girls who are trying out their new looks and methods of communicating non-verbally need all the help they can get in learning when, and when not, to turn on the 'charm'. Of course this is entirely dependent on the development of non-verbal interpretation which should have been happening throughout their life up to this time. If this has happened then the girls and boys will quickly learn the rules and suitable ways of communicating from a few experiences.

If the child has not accumulated adequate skills to help her make this transition to more adult situations she will really struggle to avoid communicating the wrong messages to teachers. Of course this applies to boys and female teachers and also to same-sex relationships, but for ease the situation of girls has been described because it is perhaps the most obvious.

Parents and teachers should be aware that:

- children need to have non-verbal understanding that is mature enough for them to make the correct choice of what they say and do

- adults are there to model what is acceptable and what is not, so that the children will learn how to behave as a 'grown-up'.

All adults have a responsibility to ensure that teenagers are given non-verbal and spoken messages that will benefit them and not confuse them, so that they will acquire and use behaviours appropriately in any given situation. All children need to be able to depend on their communication to help them make the right choices. In the teenage years this is especially important.

Post-16

It can be the case that children display few signs of behavioural, social, emotional or communication problems at primary or secondary school, mainly because they keep themselves to themselves and don't cause any behavioural difficulties as a result.

However, they can find secondary school more overwhelming due to the increasingly complex challenges described above.

Planning for post-16 placements needs to take account of youngsters' interpretational skills, otherwise they may be set up to fail. The consequence of this is that boys may end up on the wrong side of the law and girls become vulnerable to situations such as the following.

Case example

Natalie, with whom I worked some years ago, had reached secondary school without displaying many symptoms of communication problems, although everyone knew she had some learning difficulties. What she had learned, however, was to smile at people and say 'Yes'. This was an excellent strategy – because people thought that she understood what they were saying and went away.

Her secondary school were astounded when, having gone to her GP, Natalie's mother reported that she was taking knives to her parents at home and trying to throw her siblings out of bedroom windows. At school she was a 'model' pupil.

On assessment I found that Natalie understood very little of what was said to her. The most worrying thing was that she was in Year 10 and the post-16 plan was to send her

on a train to a local town where the college had a course that would meet her learning needs better.

My particular concern was her strategy for getting out of conversations. If she travelled on the train by herself and a man made a suggestion that was inappropriate, she wouldn't recognise it as such or wouldn't know that she shouldn't talk to strangers (she had trouble identifying the difference between people she had met and those she hadn't). She would simply have applied her strategy to get out of the conversation and would have smiled at him and said 'Yes'.

Teenage to adult conversations

As the child reaches the age of 14 or 15 – sometimes earlier – she will need to experience adult situations and behaviours. This is because adult conversations are very different from those of teenagers.

She should start to accompany her parents to adult events (if this is not happening naturally already) – Christmas drinks with the neighbours, conversations with adult members of the family when they visit, and so on. A young person who hasn't made the necessary development in her non-verbal conversational skills may avoid these situations by going up to her room and texting her friends, going on social network sites or watching TV, and so won't learn the skills associated with adult conversations. This will cause more teenage resentment and rows than should normally be the case.

She needs to know that she is no longer the centre of attention. She must be able to participate in the conversation and talk about what the adults are talking about, not about topics that only she is interested in.

CONCLUSION

This section has been about growing up as a teenager and the angst that it can cause. By the time she leaves school at about 18, a young person should be able to hold her own communicatively in whatever situation she finds herself.

We have seen that at the beginning of this period at the age of 11, when she enters secondary school, there is a sudden surge in the communication skills she has to develop. The pressures of this early situation were discussed and how the teachers' expectations could put a hidden pressure on the child to behave in a particular manner. All these things proliferate and impact on the child's ability to both understand what is being asked of her and behave as expected. The importance of friendships in helping children to overcome this difficult transition was highlighted.

I discussed the different models of secondary education and the benefits and pitfalls of these with regard to developing the child's potential for non-verbal communication. This is all problematic enough for the child, but on top of this her body is going into a period of huge change and her ability to cope with this and all the associated emotional changes is dependent on her communication skills being good and her confidence being high. Deterioration in confidence should be viewed as a warning that communication skills may not be as strong as they appear in a child. Good verbal language is not necessarily a sign that all is well with communication.

Finally, we looked at the transition from teenage conversations to adult ones and how the child needs to experience adult conversations in order to accumulate the skills necessary and become an independent and competent adult communicator.

If their non-verbal communication skills are functioning at the level appropriate for their age, then there is more likelihood that young people will enjoy these years and mature into confident and caring young adults.

■ 'ELDERS AND BETTERS'

ADULT DEVELOPMENT

8

As we saw in the teenage years, there is a great deal of development in the skills required to move from primary to secondary school and beyond. In the adult years through to the end of our lives, things are not so complicated. The only development that happens now is experiential, but that has a huge impact on our levels of happiness, relaxation and confidence for the rest of our lives.

■ IS THERE A DIFFERENCE BETWEEN MEN AND WOMEN?

Men and women have different preferences when it comes to communication and there are physiological reasons why this is the case. But that doesn't mean that all men communicate in the same way or that all women are better at conversations. There will always be a percentage of men who do develop excellent conversational skills, but for the purposes of this section I will stick with the majority position, which is that men prefer not to hold too many conversations and if they do, they keep them short.

We have seen in other sections of the book that boys have more difficulty learning non-verbal skills and this passes through to adult life. Women generally find holding conversations easier and seek out situations where they can talk to people.

However, men mainly use conversations for passing information and can find talking on the phone much harder. The introduction of texting through mobile phones has been a boon to male communication because texts are short and focused and require no non-verbal information processing.

Women find discussing details of events of great interest and as a result have more opportunity than men to pick up these adult experiential skills.

■ WHAT HAPPENS THROUGH THE AGES

Twenties and thirties

Newly arrived in his twenties following the turmoil of the teenage years, a man is likely to need a while to develop confidence in his communication. Women have been practising so hard up until this point that life is a little easier as a result.

Choice of job

Because of the difficulty men have in acquiring non-verbal conversational skills, their communicative level will determine the style of communicative situations they prefer. Men tend to become better at jobs that don't require too many conversations – in IT or as service engineers.

I have heard stories from parents of sons diagnosed with Asperger's syndrome while at school, who have shown a skill in fixing machines. They choose to go into business for themselves, working in a van, travelling from house to house fixing the boiler or doing the plumbing. This way the conversation will always be about the item they have specialised in. People will be very pleased because they can fix a troublesome piece of equipment and then they are on to the next house. There is a script that works and very few social niceties to learn. I am not saying that all men who choose to work this way are Asperger's, but it is a life choice – proportionately there are fewer male nurses or speech and language therapists. Jobs where you need to be good at spontaneous communication are generally dominated by women.

Even hairdressing, which possibly has more women than men, on the face of it looks like a more conversational type of profession. But it is a setting where you can learn to ask the 'right' questions socially – 'Are you going on holiday soon?' or 'What did your partner think about your last haircut?' Otherwise you don't need to look at the face of the person because your focus is on cutting the hair. The clients don't mind this because they want you to pay attention to what you are doing.

Forties to fifties

Many people say that their forties were the best years of their life. By this time conversational skills are peaking. Forty years of accumulated experiential information makes processing the mass of non-verbal information easier. Also in your forties you still have most of your faculties.

By the time you reach your fifties, conversations become even easier and you may become much more relaxed about talking to people. This period should be almost as good as your forties – depending on your health and fitness.

Over 60

In recent times, once you reached 60 your life began to slow down towards retirement. Nowadays there is tremendous economic and demographic pressure to continue working beyond the age of 60. Luckily this has coincided with an upturn in health and fitness in all ages. In my own family there are 90-year-olds who have the energy, fitness and vitality of 60- or 70-year-olds! And there are many more out there with a similar drive to live.

There may be a downside to all this vitality and determination, though. Because they continue to live and experience many things, especially since the advent of global TV and computers – my mother spends much time communicating with far-flung members of her family on Skype – older people receive more conversational stimulus and may find keeping up with the speed of younger conversations taxing.

Before the rapid expansion of information technology, older people lived at a slower pace of life and those communicating with them did so at this slow pace too. Perhaps all this increase in information is causing stress on their memory capacity – RAM overload.

 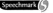

Elders research

In many societies elders are revered for their wisdom. Research has shown that the key characteristic is the ability to accurately and quickly interpret a situation, leading to successful problem solving. This is a direct result of accumulated experiential learning and a wide frame of reference with regard to non-verbal interpretation.

Dementia

In some types of dementia, perhaps the earliest symptom and one which is often missed is that the person starts to find some aspects of conversation difficult. They might start to absent themselves from large groups at family parties, or take a walk round the garden to avoid having to engage in dialogue.

There is a real similarity between the communicative changes in dementia and the development of non-verbal communication in children. But this development is going backwards. Here are the similarities in the early stages of dementia. Typically, sufferers will:

- prefer one-to-one conversations

- have difficulties conversing with more than one person at a time

- have difficulties speaking with people who are unfamiliar to them

- tend to talk about what is on their mind – usually relating to past experience.

It is therefore possible to diagnose dementia earlier through looking at people's non-verbal communication skills.

CONCLUSION

There is no need to worry about the continued development of non-verbal skills in adult life as long as the foundation skills are established in your early years. All adults really need to do communicatively is sit back and enjoy the progress into easier interpretation and information-giving.

However, it is interesting to analyse the different types of jobs that we choose to do to see whether or not conversations are at the centre. With the advent of personal computing, most of us spend a great deal of time working at a computer, which takes away time that we could be spending sharing information with friends and neighbours. These conversations might seem lightweight but they continue to polish our skills.

▪ WHAT'S MADE HIM BEHAVE LIKE THAT? ▪

PROBLEMS ASSOCIATED WITH POOR NON-VERBAL COMMUNICATION

9

Now we have seen how all these skills develop throughout our lives, in this section I will cover the problems experienced by children who fail to develop the essential non-verbal communication skills.

Conversations are central to the way we live our lives: we share information with others all day long and if we're unable to do so effectively it will impact on any or all of the following areas:

- communication of ideas and information

- emotional understanding and communication

- play and socialisation

- educational progress and career development

- confidence and self-esteem.

A child who lacks essential non-verbal conversational skills will be lost and confused with low levels of confidence, leading to poor self-esteem and having few if any friends. In this section you will see what happens when children are unable to participate in conversations from a position of strength.

Children can have non-verbal communication problems whether or not they are able to speak. This section will first look at the problems associated with those children who can speak or only choose to speak under certain circumstances, and then at those children who do not speak at all. It also covers the particular difficulties experienced by children with poorly developed skills in some or all of the key aspects of communication.

▪ DIFFICULTY WITH CONVERSATIONAL SKILLS

As the conversational skills have been covered in the sections on normal development, they will only be touched on briefly here, so please refer back for any points that need clarification.

When you encounter a behavioural, social or emotional problem in a child, first look for difficulties with conversational skills. Below are signs you will typically find in such children and which affect their behaviour, socialisation, educational attainment and emotional expression and understanding. Be aware that any child under six (or older if the problem has worsened), who is not looking at you when talking or listening, should be investigated for a non-verbal communication problem.

Listener role

The listener role is the paramount skill to develop in a child. A child who is able to listen effectively will be watching what the speaker does and learning at the same time what he needs to do to be a competent speaker.

A child must be able to do the three basic elements that are the essential prerequisite of being a good listener. If he is unable to do so he will find great difficulty in accumulating sufficient information and positive experience to help his interpretational skills – which are also a major part of good communication. He must learn to:

1 look at the speaker

2 keep still

3 listen.

Once the child has developed these first three skills as a listener, he may need to work on higher-level listener skills, such as showing interest, and also the ability to feed back to the listener if he is confused or needs clarification, for instance.

A child who has failed to develop adequate skills as a listener will commonly display evidence of the following difficulties:

- He won't look at people sufficiently between the ages of birth and primary school entry. If he is not looking at the speaker in Years 1 and 2 then he is not a good listener – never assume that he is just choosing not to look at you.

This failure to look at people sufficiently has a big impact on the child's use of his experiential knowledge to make good sense of future situations. A child who doesn't look carefully is also vulnerable to not knowing the vocabulary associated with everyday tasks, such as washing up or getting ready for school, because if he doesn't look at objects he will be unable to associate the words that go with those objects. I have worked with junior and senior pupils who have great gaps in their vocabulary for this reason.

- He will not keep still – all the children who have come for the Not Just Talking intervention had difficulty keeping still. However, even those who looked as though they had Attention Deficit and Hyperactivity Disorder (ADHD) left the intervention able to keep still and focus on conversations and on classroom lessons too – hence the improvement in their educational attainment.

- He will not listen well – he will talk about something completely unconnected with what you might be asking or saying; he will not realise that a conversation is sharing information between the two of you and so will tell you what is uppermost in his mind.

- He will learn to talk without looking at the person he is speaking to.

These problems are all associated directly with poor listener skills. Here are a couple of cases to help illustrate some poor listener skills:

Case examples

When I first saw Max he just couldn't sit still or be still. He was full of energy and described by his parents as a 'handful', and the school found he needed too much support to focus on his school work. He was big for his age – six-and-a-half – and tended to bound up to other children in the playground, knocking them over in the process. For the first four intervention sessions I worked on sitting still with him, but began to think that this child was going to be the first one not to be able to do so. However, I persevered. Suddenly in the sixth session there was a major breakthrough: he came in and sat still for 80 per cent of the session! This had also transferred to his classroom behaviour and he started to get rewards for being helpful in class and in the playground.

There are only a few children who have been referred to Not Just Talking who did not have a difficulty with looking at people. One sticks out in my mind, though, because his parents had obviously heard that 'eye contact' was important. So when I first went to assess Joseph, I observed him with his class on the mat listening to the teacher. By about 10–15 minutes into the session, the other children were beginning to wriggle and fidget, but Joseph kept on looking at the teacher. In the end he was the only one still looking at her. When the session was over, I took him in for assessment and the first thing I asked was 'What was your teacher talking about?' He looked at me quizzically as though I was slightly mad to ask such a thing and then said 'I don't know'. Joseph had no idea what had been said. Probably if I had asked a few of his peers who hadn't been looking at the teacher, they would have been able to give me some ideas of what she was talking about.

In Freaks, *Geeks and Asperger Syndrome: A User Guide to Adolescence*, Luke Jackson (2003) tells others who have been diagnosed with Asperger's syndrome not to make eye contact but to look at people's mouths. He says he finds this easier, although more distracting because the mouth moves so much. This is an Asperger's lad advising other Asperger's children about how to give the impression that you are looking at people – as they wish – but also demonstrating that he has no idea why we do this. In my experience, even children diagnosed with Asperger's syndrome can learn how to develop the non-verbal interpretation skills that I advocate in this book, and once they know why they are looking at people they do it without even having to think about it.

An important way to help a child is not to ask him to 'give eye contact'. Also, only ask him to look at you when he has sufficient skills to process the information he can see. Otherwise, like Joseph in the examples above, he will look and still be none the wiser about the topic of conversation because he won't know that the purpose of looking at faces is to read expressions, not to simply to make eye contact.

Speaker role

It is the speaker's job to deliver the message in a suitable manner so that it can be received and understood by the listener – whether in a one-to-one situation or in small or large groups.

A child with low ability in this area of conversational skills will either talk about topics that he is confident with, such as dinosaurs or fantasy games; or he will shut down, by opting out of conversations. Because he is unable to understand the supplementary questions in a dialogue he determines what he will talk about and for how long.

His conversational performance will vary as a result because in some situations – generally one-to-one with people he knows well – he is able to cope with questions about topics he is well versed in. But in other situations with small groups of peers or with adults he is not familiar with, he will revert to trying to talk about his favourite topic, ignoring what the other person is interested in or needs to know.

I have come to realise that the latter behaviour can be seen in elective and selective mutes. The fact that they either choose to speak to certain people and not others or opt out completely is exactly the same as the children with behavioural difficulties who do this. Therefore, in theory, children who fall under this diagnosis should respond to the Not Just Talking intervention method.

Any child who dominates the conversation as a speaker or opts out will not have learned to be a 'good' speaker and will demonstrate some of the following difficulties:

Case example

Alex was referred by his parents when he was nine years old. He had a history of poor language development but when he finally started talking he was described as having a 'sing-song' voice and 'weird quirks'. He had been diagnosed as having Asperger's syndrome.

Assessment

On assessment his communication problem was so severe that he was unable to give information if asked specific questions, and under these circumstances he would be hesitant and his sentence length would be very short. However, when he was able to turn the conversation round to his preferred topics, his sentence length suddenly increased and the confidence in his voice was quite evident. Once on his topic, though, it was hard to redirect him.

For the teacher in his mainstream primary class, this variation in Alex's communication – from hardly anything to far too much – was hard to predict and handle. Before assessment no one fully understood the depth of his communication difficulty and the implications for him – see www.notjusttalking.co.uk where his mother talks of her relief at learning about the non-verbal communication problems he had so that she could help him communicate more effectively.

Alex's strategy to help him deal with his poor interpretational skills was to tell you all

about his fantasies (see behaviour section below for more on strategies). He liked planning computer games as this was a favourite activity for him at home. He has a younger brother but on assessment there was little positive engagement between the two of them because Alex would suddenly explode and throw things or hit out. So his parents, as most parents do, tended to keep them apart.

Also, although he recognised some basic emotions he had no idea what had caused his feelings as he couldn't put himself in someone else's shoes and think what they were thinking – absence of theory of mind. Generally his interpretational skills were very poor.

Part of his communication problem was that he was also not a good listener, especially as he didn't look at people sufficiently. But the biggest problem that Alex experienced was that he couldn't make friends. Of course, as his communication was so limited and he was only able to give people information about topics of interest to him, this was the biggest hurdle to overcome.

After the Not Just Talking intervention

Initially we worked on improving his skills as a listener and developing his interpretation through the Not Just Talking strategy. Once these areas started to improve in the first few sessions, Alex began to be able to give information pertinent to the situation at a rudimentary level.

As the intervention progressed it became clear that, although some areas of his vocabulary concerning his preferred topics were excellent, his basic vocabulary associated with daily living was poor to non-existent.

When asked what he had been doing at school, he would only tell you what he had been thinking of during the morning – what complex game he had designed or some other fantasy that he thought up. His understanding of what was reality and what was fantasy was very blurred. But soon he learned about the difference between what happened in the 'real' world and what was in his mind and he would talk about his experiences in class and the playground. Once he was able to do this, it meant that he could learn from his experience at last.

Once he had developed theory of mind and had started to improve his information-giving skills, he began to participate in everyday activities in the home and gradually his vocabulary improved.

This happened slowly, because at first his parents weren't aware of how poor his vocabulary was and, like most parents with children approaching or older than 10 years, they tended to stick to strategies that had worked in the past to reduce the behaviour problems.

Very unusually, I decided that they should watch an intervention session – this was after over a year of sessions so I thought that Alex would not react badly. Having individually observed the difficulty that Alex had interpreting complex situations, due to his limited life experiences, Alex's parents started to engage him in everyday activities and suddenly his whole world opened up.

151

After a great deal of improvement in his communication, Alex still struggled to make friends. But a visit to school helped his mother find out what the problem was – lots of children wanted to be his friend but because of the severity of his difficulties he was unable to transfer his new communication skills to this challenging situation. With a bit more help from school – they pointed out to him that the approaches made by his classmates were because they wanted to be friends – and continued help at home, he began to overcome his difficulty and make friends.

Giving information

There is more on this subject below under 'Topic-related skills'. The ability to give information is a skill that a child has to develop early in his life. He will only be able to do this if he is a good listener and can process the non-verbal signals that help him understand what to say.

A child will find giving information under pressure very difficult and his grammatical utterances will change from well-formed phrases of usual length to maybe one- or two-word utterances. Remember that just because a child can perform well in one situation doesn't mean that he will be able to perform at the same level all the time. It is very easy for people to assume that a confident manner of talking at great length demonstrates a normal skill level. It is his hesitant one- or two-word responses that indicate his real level of communication development.

Asking for help

Another difficulty that you will see in a child is that he doesn't ask for help. This will range from not asking for practical things like help with tying his shoelaces to more complex tasks such as asking an adult to clarify an instruction or a peer to explain the rules of a game. The effect of not developing this skill follows this pattern:

1   In every conversation it is the role of the speaker to ensure that:

   • the information given is what the receiver wants or needs

   • the information is given in a manner easily understood by the listener

   • if the listener can't understand the information it is given again, but in a different way or with different words, so that the listener is able to understand.

   This is most often done in response to a look of confusion on the listener's face.

2   A child who has non-verbal communication problems and therefore hasn't looked at people sufficiently in the previous years of his life won't recognise that this is what happens during a conversation.

3   So if he hasn't learned to ask for help at a simple level, such as when he has dropped his spoon, then he will not have learned the more complex skill of asking for help during a conversation so that people can make what they're saying easier for him to understand.

4 He remains confused because he doesn't know to ask for help. So he doesn't get any help to make better sense of what is being said. It becomes a problem that is compounded in every conversation.

5 Those who hold conversations with him will think that he has understood because he hasn't asked for help. This makes them expect that he will behave in a way appropriate to the conversation.

6 It is a vicious spiral. By the time a child is seven or eight he might find himself experiencing high levels of frustration and confusion or alienation as a result of not asking for help in the course of an exchange.

7 Also he won't have any idea that everyone else can be confused about what is said to them as he can't recognise the non-verbal or verbal clues through which others ask for help.

So it is vital that parents make sure their child has the confidence and ability to ask for help. Later in life there will be many situations where this skill will be of use: from understanding a maths problem, to learning to ride a bike, to dealing with emotions, and so on.

Negotiation

The ability to negotiate depends directly on the effectiveness of your conversational skills; a child who has difficulty in this area is extremely vulnerable in the playground because in any situation of conflict that arises he will be unable to placate his peers. Such children should not be left alone with their peers to resolve difficult situations as they will be unable to do so until their conversational skills improve.

Styles of conversation

Remember that if a child is talking to everyone in the same manner this is a good indication of a serious non-verbal communication difficulty and suggests that the child should be assessed. By the time a child enters primary school, he should at least be able to talk in different styles to his parents, his siblings, his teachers, his peers and strangers.

Topic-related skills

There are quite a few skills that come under this heading and for ease I will deal with each one separately. However, they all have two things in common – their use is dependent on non-verbal interpretation and understanding, and it is easy to spot when a child lacks skill in these areas.

Initiating topics

A child who is unable to initiate a topic is quite often described as 'attention seeking'. This is because, while he is able to approach people, when he gets there he doesn't have the skill of initiating a conversation so will 'hang around' or become disruptive.

This might seem a simple act but in fact starting a conversation off is quite a hard thing to do.

1 First you need to know that it is your turn to talk (see below for the complexity of this skill).

2 Next you need to know the openers for a conversation. A child who can't say 'Excuse me' or 'Hello, how are you?' or 'Can I go to the toilet?' (or versions which use fewer words) will be unable to get the conversation going.

3 He must understand the need to have a message to give. As he is unlikely to appreciate that you don't already know what is in his mind, he won't realise that he needs to give you information in the first place.

Topic choosing

Initiating leads directly into the next skill – choosing a topic. If a child chooses a topic that is of interest only to him this demonstrates that he has poor interpretational and prediction skills because he is unable to judge what is a suitable topic for the situation. He will have to be able to read the information available from the person/people present, relate that to the situation and his past experience and then choose the topic that is most appropriate. It could be a topic of his choice, as he needs to ask a question, but he also needs to develop the skill of selecting a topic based on his understanding of the non-verbal clues given by the people and situation. So a child who is able to do all this is unlikely to have a non-verbal communication difficulty.

Topic maintenance

'Topic maintenance' means being able to keep a topic going for the requisite period of time – not too long or too little. Problems with topic maintenance are very clear because a child who is unable to do this will talk a great deal about the things that fascinate him and will, in difficult situations, give very little information when asked direct questions that need a clear response, for example, 'How many brothers and sisters have you got?'

The reason why a child sticks to topics he knows is best explained by looking at adult conversational performance in different situations. Think of a topic that you know a great deal about, such as cooking or fixing cars or paper folding, or anything job-related that you have developed some sort of expertise in. I would suggest that if asked to talk to a small group of five or less about this topic you would be able to do so, and probably with confidence. Initially you might dread it, but because you are experienced and knowledgeable about the topic you could do it, and the more you spoke the more your confidence would grow.

However, if the next talk was to a much larger group with little time to prepare, about a topic that you had little or no knowledge of, then your confidence level would be low and you would find the task so challenging that you might seek to avoid it. What has happened here is that the stress factors have increased: first, there are more people in the audience and second, you will feel less confident about the topic. Being exposed in this way would reduce your fluency and might cause you to adopt behaviours such as avoidance or deflection – reactions you might recognise in children.

A child talks about his topic of interest because he knows and likes it and has a large vocabulary to draw on. He has practised it on many occasions and talking about this topic gives him confidence. This is completely the opposite to his experience of other situations where people ask him for information about topics he is not so familiar with. At these times he will either dominate the conversation with a subject that makes him feel confident and successful, thereby avoiding the subjects making him feel panicky and stressed, or he may deflect the conversation, respond in one- or two-word utterances or simply opt out altogether.

Turn to talk

The vast majority of the signals telling you when it is your turn to talk are non-verbal. So it goes without saying that children with poor skills in this area will not know about taking turns in conversations. In fact, they rarely know what the purpose of a conversation is, so do not be surprised if they interrupt or dominate. Playing board games, however, is not a good remedy for poor turn-taking skills. These signals are associated with both aural and visual perception and are more subtle than can be easily demonstrated by participating in a game.

Ending the topic

Knowing when to end a topic depends on the speaker looking at the listener so that it is clear when the listener has heard enough information or needs some clarification. Children with non-verbal communication difficulties don't look at the listener, and even if they do they can't read the facial expressions that communicate messages of this kind. So you will come across children who talk for far too long and find it very hard to change topic as a result. These children also struggle to know when someone else is about to stop talking, so tend to butt in.

Topic appropriateness

Knowing which topics might be appropriate for the person and situation depends on our processing skills, drawing on the non-verbal information available. If we get this right and can predict what the conversation needs to be about and use our shared knowledge appropriately, then we are more likely to identify a suitable topic. However, a child with poor interpretational skills will struggle with this and may well say some inappropriate things as a result. Here are a few examples from my experience of assessment and the initial information given about the child:

- 'That baby is going to eat the dog!'

- A child who wrote a card for another child in his class who had been very ill and said 'I hope that you never get better'.

- Looking at a picture of a nurse putting a sling on a girl's arm, I have been told, quite a few times, that the girl was being sick and the nurse was catching the sick in a tea cloth.

This ability to keep things appropriate is of course much more taxing when in group settings, which is why assembly is so difficult for children who are unable to process the non-verbal signals telling them what can and cannot be said and when to keep quiet.

POOR INTERPRETATIONAL SKILLS

In order to be able to interpret well, we all have to be good at being able to:

1 'read' facial expressions and body language – two separate but related areas – to pick up messages

2 take in the situation or context

3 compare what you see and hear with your experience of similar situations.

Only if we use these three sources of information and knowledge equally will our interpretation of what is to be said or done be accurate.

Once this interpretation is made we then have to select from maybe two or three options which behaviour or communication technique to use. Here is an example to help illustrate this point.

You see a lot of people congregating in a large area. They are waiting to go into another room. From their clothes you realise that they are very smartly dressed and it is daytime. Their communication to each other and their body language tells you that they are anticipating someone's arrival.

You recognise the room as being part of a church because of your experience of other churches.

With this information your experience tells you that it might be a funeral or a wedding or, if it is Sunday, it might just be people going to church. However, the clothes tip the balance towards a wedding because they are more colourful than you would see at a funeral and smarter than people would normally wear to church.

Now you know what is going on and if you talk to these people, you might say something like 'Whose wedding is it?' But if it was a service on a Sunday morning the question might be 'Which hymn are we singing?'

The difficulty that you will witness in a child with poor non-verbal skills is that he might do any or a combination of the following:

- misinterpret the body language – he will not pick up on what the clothes or body language communicate

- not recognise the situation – if he looks at the books on sale he might think it's a shop and not the ante-chamber of a church

- his experience being limited, he might think that the people were there to buy comics – because that is what he likes to do at a book/papershop.

There are more examples of misinterpretation in the Section 11 on the assessment of non-verbal communication difficulties.

Level of interpretation

A child might be able to recognise a few emotions but this is not sufficient on its own. Not only will he need to learn to be able to read many different emotions: at least 30 (see examples below) but he also needs to recognise the different levels at which we communicate emotions.

Possible emotions that children should learn (this is not an exhaustive list and may vary from child to child):

Happy	Surprised	Worried	Unsure	Confused
Sad	Love	Dislike	Smug	Disinterested
Angry	Want	Bored	Afraid	Focus
Interested	Scared	Unfriendly	Lonely	Fond
Jealous	Moody	Secretive	Unsure	Shocked
Kind	Upset	Hurt	Smug	Thoughtful
Pleased	Friendly	Like	Shy	Pleased

There are many levels, but at the early stages of learning this skill he would just need level 1, 2 and 3.

Making sense of information

Another problem for these children is that they don't use information given by others to make better sense of what is going on. This is partly due to their interpretational difficulties and partly because they have not learned to ask for help in a conversation.

Making good sense of a verbal message depends on non-verbal interpretation. Because a child with poor interpretational skills is listening to every word said to him, the words build up like a train in a tunnel with no exit. Eventually he will be totally overloaded with information that he can't process and then his strategies will kick in. He will do all he can to get out of the conversation that has made him so confused. See Section 6 for guidance on how to handle this.

Difficulties with interpretation signals

Signs that a child is finding interpretation difficult include all the reactions described in 'problems associated with behaviour' below. He will start to behave in a manner which is suddenly and unexpectedly different from how he has been behaving and, if people continue to talk to him at this juncture, his behaviour will deteriorate. He must be left on his own to recuperate – only he can bring himself back from this confused state.

Experiential learning

The development of a child's 'database' of experiential information is based on his ability to process non-verbal information as it occurs and to store it to be used at a later date for the purpose of making comparisons and drawing conclusions. Children with poor interpretational skills do not have access to all the information experienced throughout their childhood and, because their range of experience is also limited, the store of information available to them on a moment-to-moment basis is significantly reduced.

Those children who have good verbal understanding and expression combined with good interpretational skills will accumulate a wealth of information that helps them to process situational information well and leads to good understanding and communication.

Hidden meanings

Being able to understand metaphors usually starts quite early in a child's life. James Geary (2011) reports in his book *I is an Other* that Dedre Gentner had found a sliding scale of increasingly complex similes to test children aged five through to teenagers. She found that physical similarities developed first but that similes that related to feelings developed much later. Geary also says that children's spoken language is full of metaphor because they often can't think of the right word so might come up with combinations to make what he calls 'kennings'. For example, my children often described things using kennings: a local department store called 'Tyrrell & Greens' was where we went for curtain material – to our children it became known as 'material greens'! It is still called that in our family today. A simpler use of metaphors was when they referred to broccoli as 'trees'.

A child who is unable to understand hidden meanings will interpret what he hears literally, so will react to phrases such as 'don't blow your top' or 'you really take the biscuit' in a manner completely differently from what is expected.

Another problem you may notice is that the child has great difficulty understanding verbal jokes. He might well understand visual humour but because verbal jokes depend on being able to interpret hidden meanings, children with non-verbal communication difficulties can't do this.

Finally, he will not understand sarcasm. This is because of the conflict between the verbal message, facial expression and body language. Children will react only to the verbal message, such as 'you'd forget your head if it wasn't screwed on', so will be mystified by what the teacher is saying.

COGNITIVE SKILLS

Cognitive skills, such as the ability to predict, draw conclusions and make connections between information and situations, are an essential tool of communication and help the child to select appropriate communication and behaviour for the people and the situation. The lack of these skills is demonstrated in the following ways. (I will also cover the effect of things done by others in the child's environment.)

Prediction

A child who cannot predict is very noticeable and vulnerable at school. He will see his teacher get out a book and sit down in front of the class who are all sitting still on a mat, but he will fail to predict what the teacher is going to do – read a story – even though he may have seen this activity many times before. Those who can predict will know what to do but those who can't may well do something completely inappropriate.

Also, a child may be unable to predict the consequences of his actions. So when told by other children to do something like pull a chair from under another child, he won't understand the consequence or the possibility of injuring the child, and so is more likely to do it.

These children are very vulnerable to being 'wound up' by others to do things that they wouldn't dare to do themselves, and they are often the ones who are admonished or excluded as a result of the action. The other children, despite their part in knowingly provoking the child, often get away scot-free.

Case example

One case I remember was of Raymond, who had a reputation as a younger child (at KS2 and the start of KS3) for saying things to girls and to teachers that were totally unacceptable, such as 'I want to punch your teeth in to see the blood running'. This particular phrase was the result of his playing 'Mortal Combat'. If you look at what happens in that game, the fighters literally do that.

The reason that he was playing such games on his computer was because of his communication problem (see 'TV/screens' at the end of this section). And having seen this happen on a screen where the characters got up afterwards and continued fighting, he had no idea that punching someone would hurt them.

It was when he became a large teenager that saying these words became really menacing. At this stage, though, he never followed through with the physical violence. However, people's collective impression of him was that he was dangerous and might hit out at you. This stuck to him even when his behaviour had improved and it followed him round in situations in school as part of his 'story'.

The difficulty for him was that just saying this to a small female teacher, made her feel scared and intimidated. She truly believed that he would follow through and hurt her. Understandably, he was excluded.

Another part of Ray's history that went everywhere with him was that he had been accused at around the age of 11 of saying that he wanted to rape a girl in his year. It is more than likely that he had no idea what he was talking about at that stage. But because it was reported by the girl to the teacher he was excluded.

Later, when his conversational skills improved, though not sufficiently to cope in difficult situations where he lost his temper, he was wound up either knowingly or unknowingly by the girl who had accused him two or three years earlier. His perception was that she was following him round and, despite his best efforts to avoid her in the school, he would bump into her when moving from class to class. He saw this as her choosing to meet him. On these occasions there would be much laughter from the girl which was interpreted by Ray as her laughing at him, rather than her being nervous, which she probably was.

During one of these occasions there was some conflict between them and the girl accused Ray of repeating the phrase that he had said two or three years earlier, 'I am going to rape you'. Ray totally denied this – which may or may not have been true – but in reality the situation was a combination of the girl not keeping away from this boy and his lack of complete understanding of her intentions. She didn't do what she had been asked by the teachers to do, which was to keep away from him. Simply by being in the wrong place at the wrong time she caused Ray to do or say something that he probably didn't mean to say.

The impact on Ray was a more 'permanent' exclusion. At this point, I recommended removal from the school. This was just due to the fact that most people in the school saw Ray as a boy who said things that made people feel very vulnerable.

Ray moved to another school in another town, and there were absolutely no problems. In fact, the school said that they didn't recognise the boy described in the paperwork that accompanied his transfer.

So being able to predict has an important bearing on many types of behaviour – Ray was unable to predict the reaction of people to what he said and so was surprised by the outcome. I have spent most of my time while working with these children in trying to advocate for them. It seems completely wrong that children with special needs are excluded and the children who have provoked them to react in ways that lead to exclusion are able to remain in the system.

Drawing conclusions

At school, it is expected that a child has this skill. He will need to make inferences not only from what is going on in the class and playground but also from what he has read. Without the basic ability to draw conclusions he will be unable to apply this skill to reading. If children can't draw conclusions they may learn to read but not understand what they are reading.

Teachers should check that the child is able to infer from a situation. For instance, if a picture shows a family of two children and a mother going towards a farm which sells tickets to go and visit the animals, can the child tell that they are going into the entrance of the farm? Does the child know what they are about to do? Buy tickets?

If the child is only able to describe the situation – there is a mum and a girl and a boy, or there is another woman inside the building – they are at an earlier stage of communicative development and will need intervention to develop the ability to draw conclusions. If the child can only describe, then the teacher should not attempt to teach the child to read and expect him to do so with meaning.

Lack of structure

As we have seen in the sections on normal development, structure is very important to help children know what is going on and what is about to happen next. This is why timetables have become so popular with autistic children. However, personal timetables on the child's desk are important for all children with poor prediction skills.

A child should be given as much support as necessary to help him to identify the beginnings and ends of activities until he is able to recognise boundaries without support.

Connections leading to generalisation

The ability to make connections – to cross-reference information from one situation to another – is both a central communication skill as well as one that will enable a child to reach his full educational potential.

Evidence of no connections

Look for children who can't apply knowledge gained in one situation to another. This is fairly evident with children who have a learning disability, but may be harder to recognise in children who can talk well. Then the most likely indicator is that the child may be able to talk about how to get ready for PE in a situation where all the children are doing so, but would be unable to describe it later in the day when something else such as numeracy is going on.

Children I work with typically see only some of the information or need help to interpret what they see in one picture of a sequence. When shown the next picture they are quite unable to make use of information gained from the previous picture to make a good interpretation of the next picture.

Generalisation

This ability to connect information is a skill that underpins our capacity to generalise from one situation to another. Children on the autistic spectrum are deemed unable to develop the skill of generalisation. But when you read Section 12 on the Not Just Talking intervention method you will find that one of the main outcomes of the intervention – even for children on the autistic spectrum – is that they learn to generalise.

Conforming to rules/norms

A child who has not developed the ability to generalise effectively will be unable to use information to generate rules that work for him in different situations – including apparent exceptions. So he is likely to apply a rule that is deemed 'bizarre' by others, especially teachers. Suppose a child goes into a chemistry lab at school and takes out the Bunsen burner ready for his chemistry lesson. The rule he is applying may well have been acquired during a previous chemistry lesson, but he has not picked up other clues which indicate that this is actually an English lesson but the only room available was the laboratory. Consequently he applied the wrong rule. The rule would also have been wrong if it had been a chemistry lesson but the teacher was covering another topic that day which didn't include the use of Bunsen burners.

This is not just a matter of listening to what he is told but also requires him to register and interpret a range of visual, aural and contextual evidence over a period of time and to make the necessary connections.

A child might also pick up the wrong rule from his peers, and may well apply the rule in a situation where his teacher is expecting behaviour of another kind. This will set the child up to come into conflict with his teacher which, again, he may not be able to resolve because of his poor conversational skill development.

Of course, on entry to school, particularly secondary school, there are many 'rules' or behaviours which differ according to the teacher, place and subject, so a child who is struggling with a limited number of rules to apply is at a great disadvantage. There is more about the rules a child needs to learn in Sections 6 and 7.

EMOTIONAL IMPACT

Poor interpretational skills impact on the child's ability to understand emotion in others or communicate non-verbally about his own feelings and emotions.

Limited range of understanding and expression

A consequence of poor understanding of body language and facial expressions is that a child will be unable to use these forms of communication himself because he doesn't understand what they mean or how the feelings have been caused. The child may feel emotions welling up in him, but will not be able to attribute the cause or name the emotion because these connections were not made in the period between birth and school entry.

Such a child is likely to only notice extreme expressions of emotion and can only use the emotions he sees, so he notices anger only when the person is in a rage and shouting at him. As a result, when he becomes angry he communicates at this same high level. He has never learned to notice the lower levels of anger because they were too subtle.

This is why I have often been told that the referred child 'appears to explode with anger for no apparent reason'. People are confused because the level of emotion does not match the trigger event. If people just asked what had made the child angry, they would learn that the cause was something very simple, like breaking a pencil lead or another child pulling his clothes. The anger displayed by the child would be the same if something more serious had happened, because he only has one emotional 'gear', as it were.

Also, the child will not recognise that different people communicate feelings and degrees of feelings in slightly different ways. Because he hasn't picked up the subtler methods of communicating emotions, it is likely that he won't recognise these variations. This of course is often not helped by the fact that he doesn't look at faces sufficiently.

Remember that a child must first learn to understand emotions in order to be able to communicate his own feelings effectively.

Complex emotional understanding

As a child reaches his teens a lack of emotional understanding leads to a state of confusion and stress. Children are very vulnerable to depression at this age, either from not understanding what is happening to them or from having to keep up with the increased complexity of emotions being communicated to them by peers and adults.

Children will become isolated and may get involved with gangs or other kids whose communication development is not as good as it needs to be at this age. Teenagers are very vulnerable and those who have non-verbal processing difficulties are often the ones who end up getting into trouble. As we have seen, this is often a result of their poor prediction skills impairing their ability to anticipate the likely outcome of behaviour in which they have been encouraged by their peer group.

PROBLEMS ASSOCIATED WITH BEHAVIOUR

When a child behaves in a way that is deemed inappropriate, people should ask the question 'What has made him behave like that?' As we saw earlier in this section, the result of a child not being able to process the vast amount of non-verbal information bombarding his brain is to send it into overload and confusion. The child will then adopt strategies to get out of the confused situation. Initially these are fairly innocuous, but if he is not listened to then the behaviours become increasingly challenging and result in physical aggression. The idea is to stop his behaviour from escalating by using the strategies recommended – see point 12 under 'Mixed-ability classes: strategies to use in class' in Section 6.

What happens if people keep talking?

When a child has gone into this state of confusion, only he can bring himself back to 'normal' functioning. Talking to him at this stage is like pouring petrol on a fire: it will only inflame his feelings of frustration and impotence. In fact, many parents, despite not understanding the reason why, will adopt the tactic of sending the child to his room, knowing that if he stays with the family his behaviour will escalate.

During the Not Just Talking intervention, parents often hang on to the tactics that worked for them in the past beyond the time when the child needs them. It is a pleasant surprise when they realise that the child is happy to engage with them at the meal table.

What strategies do children adopt?

Children use these strategies to get out of conversations. Often a child will say quite clearly what it is that he wants you to do, for instance I have often heard children say to adults, 'Stop talking to me'. If you do not listen to these signals from the child, his behaviour will deteriorate and may develop in any of the ways described below.

The child may adopt a particular behaviour or a combination of behaviours according to the severity of his non-verbal confusion. A child who shows any of the following signs should be investigated for non-verbal communication difficulties before any other diagnosis or treatment – such as medication – is tried.

Inappropriate verbal language

At a low level, the child might just start using inappropriate words such as swear words that he has picked up without knowing their full meaning. However, he might start to understand the impact and use them more often as a result. This phase may mingle with the next strategy of verbal dominance.

Verbal dominance

A child will just want to dominate the conversation by talking non-stop about his topic of interest. This is beneficial to him because he is in control as the 'giver' of information and if he talks a great deal there is little opportunity for his listener to ask him awkward questions that he can't answer.

This domination of the conversation continues until the child develops good non-verbal interpretational skills which allow him to deal effectively with what other people are saying to him.

Verbal aggression

If people do not understand why the first two strategies are being used and continue to talk to the child – even for the best of motives – then he is likely to become verbally abusive or aggressive. This is simply an attempt to deflect or stop the conversation. Remember, once confused, the child himself is the only person who can rescue him from that state and this can only be done when no one else is talking to him.

Physical aggression

If the signals are really not recognised or the child is severely confused, then he will feel powerless and is likely to resort to violent behaviour, either hitting out at others or throwing objects.

Another factor of the child's difficulty with non-verbal interpretation is that he may not understand that if he hits others, they feel pain. This is due to his lack of 'theory of mind' – if he hits someone he will at best think the person feels the same as he does, ie, not much pain, so he may appear surprised at their reaction.

The more physically aggressive the child becomes, the more likely he is to be excluded from school. It is at this point that these children start to really cost local authorities a great deal of money. All this could be avoided by these children receiving intervention at an early age.

Opt out

These last two strategies are not generally accompanied by physical aggression unless the child is not listened to over a protracted period. A child who becomes so confused and frustrated that he cannot cope might just shut down and not communicate at all with anyone. Here is an example from my caseload of a child who was having a great problem because he chose not to talk to people.

Case example

David had found primary school so difficult that there were many periods in his life when he just stayed at home. All sorts of services were engaged as a result of this 'unauthorised' absence from school, but on his return he would avoid contact and most often would be found either with his hood over his face – blocking out others – or under the stage, where adults found it hard to access him as the space was too small.

At any sign of communicative or academic pressure he would opt out of the situation, and if people didn't listen he would use physical aggression to get his way. He constantly wore his coat in school so that he could hide behind his hood if the situation arose. The only way that the school had found to work with him at all was in a small room between classrooms where he could be on his own.

David's behaviour had resulted in him missing out on so much education that he was kept in primary school for an extra year. This also gave an opportunity for children's services to agree an appropriate secondary placement with his mother.

It was only at this time that Not Just Talking became involved. On assessment it was obvious how problematic communication was for this boy, but because he had 'boxed' himself into a world that he could cope with for so long, he was not open to direct work on his communication.

A programme was devised using Not Just Talking methods to enable David to participate in the activities. He had a learning support assistant trained and advised by me for five mornings a week. By working with him in this way, we got him to participate in a small programme of activities for the morning. Until this point in time it was hit or miss whether David would participate in anything while at school.

It was agreed with the school that his 'space' would not be used as a transit route while he was working there. This would only have served to distract David from his programme and add confusing non-verbal signals that he would find too hard to process.

He learned to choose appropriately what would be on the timetable and gradually, as his choosing skills improved, he accepted 'curriculum' subjects being part of this plan. However, the timetable was flexible and didn't require long periods of time doing one thing.

He soon stopped wearing his coat except when passing through the busy areas of the school. He started attending swimming (which was an activity he really enjoyed but couldn't participate in because of all the other children.)

His mother really noticed a difference in him. For years he had been a cause of such worry to her as he found everything so hard. She reported that he had started engaging with the children in the playground while waiting for his brother to come out of school, and he asked her questions about what she was thinking for the first time in his life.

The Not Just Talking contract was only for the time he stayed at the primary school and this move happened at the end of the academic year.

My recommendations for David were that he would still find working in a class very hard and a big change of location would be detrimental, but he couldn't stay where he was so he moved on. Unfortunately this placement did not last long and this resulted in him having to be supported at home.

This example shows that:

- some children find processing non-verbal information very difficult, and as a result they have to protect themselves from confusion and confrontation because they don't have the conversational skills to deal with either of these

- a child who has 'boxed himself in' so much finds making the move to secondary school virtually impossible.

Flight

Finally, for all the reasons already discussed, a child might decide that running away from the situation is the best option to avoid those who are talking to him. This is a very dangerous strategy which challenges any school that has to deal with such a child. Here is a short case history of a child who was unable to predict and as a result would flee from the school.

Case example

This boy, John, was a Year 5 child who would flee from his class if he knew that someone he didn't know was coming to see him. This was a result of his very poor interpretational skills, which meant that he couldn't predict on the following levels:

1 *He had no idea what the person might be going to do or what they might be going to say. So rather than stay around to be made to feel confused, he would leave before the situation arose.*

2 *Until his predictive skills improved he could not use his past experience of situations. This would have helped him to know that if his mother and the class teacher wanted him to see a person, nothing bad would happen.*

The main difficulty was that next term John was going to secondary school. Not Just Talking's programme would have helped, but maybe not at this late stage. My concern was how a secondary school would deal with a child who fled from class and school at the first sign of trouble. Things deteriorated for John in Year 6 and he didn't last long in mainstream secondary school. He is now in specialist provision.

As you will see from all these strategies, basically all the child is trying to do is escape his confusion. However, seen from others' point of view, the child's behaviour is inappropriate and may be attention seeking; at secondary school children are often called 'malicious' or some other interpretation – with the connotation that they are deliberately choosing to act in a certain way.

Use of medication

One of the most frustrating aspects of my work with children is that quite often, before their communication difficulty is addressed, medication is prescribed to deal with the behaviours, attention problems and perceived hyperactivity.

The Not Just Talking intervention method addresses the behaviour and fidgeting in one-to-one sessions over a 12-week period without the need for medication – surely a better route to take?

Tantrums

Tantrums beyond the usual expected age of two or three are a sign that the child's non-verbal interpretation skills are not keeping pace with his verbal language development. I have witnessed 14-year-olds lying on the floor kicking and screaming because they have not understood what is going to happen to them. So any child who continues to throw tantrums should be investigated for signs of non-verbal communication difficulties.

EDUCATIONAL IMPACT

We have seen elsewhere in this book that children's behaviour can vary from home to school, ie, they can be badly behaved at home but not at school and vice versa. This is accounted for by the following factors found in the school or home setting:

What promotes good behaviour?	What promotes poor behaviour?
Single child	The lack of structure in home life
The level of structure inherent in school life	Sibling rivalry
Child's desire to hold himself 'tight' and not display poor behaviour	Competition from peers when trying to form friendships
	Change in teachers – styles and expectations
	Child tired when gets home so 'lets go'

So now let's look at the impact on behaviour of other aspects of a child's education and the expectations of the current educational system in the UK.

The impact of non-verbal conversational problems on education

Currently the level of disruption caused on a personal level, at class level and at whole school level by the poor behaviour resulting from inadequate non-verbal conversational skill is a huge issue for many schools. The strategies and behaviours adopted by these children contribute directly to the following problems in schools:

- children not reaching their potential, either because they are not able to follow lessons because of their communication difficulty, or because the behaviour of those children with poor non-verbal communication skills distracts others in the class

- children's aggressive behaviour in class and the playground

- social adjustment difficulties in and out of school

- children who are excluded from school either temporarily or permanently.

The full cost to society in terms of impact on both family/carers and the child has not been calculated, but encompasses:

- the consequences of family breakdown

- the frustration of all staff who work with these children – who end up feeling exhausted, deskilled and frustrated as they go round in circles trying the same approaches but never changing the child's behaviour, and the potential impact on teacher retention

- the high cost of 'out-of-county' placements and the impact on children's services' budgets

- anti-social behaviour and the impact on old and young

- the cost to the police and judicial services of dealing with the consequences of poor social adjustment

- the opportunity costs of young people failing to achieve their individual academic and career potential.

When balanced against the cost of early intervention – or prevention – such as Not Just Talking's programmes, it is evident that huge savings could be made – and far more children could be equipped to live more fulfilling lives.

Return from school

Parents know that all children come back from school exhausted and need a while to 'wind down'. They soon learn that it is best to leave the child alone with a snack to calm down, usually in front of the TV, before making too many demands on him. Here are some reasons why the behaviour of a child with non-verbal communication difficulties suddenly deteriorates on getting home:

- He is exhausted after a long day at school where he has been trying hard to contain outbursts of behaviour.

 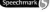

- He will have been very stressed, impotent or alienated in certain situations, but if he has contained himself he will have used up all his energy.

- Siblings may be making demands on the parents and a child who lacks interpretational skills can't understand why he is not the centre of attention, so this might set him on a path of deteriorating behaviour.

- Children have been known to attack their siblings as a result of confusion or misinterpretation.

- Academic or social pressures – such as rushing out to after-school activities or lots of homework to complete – will exacerbate the child's problems in knowing what is happening or going to happen. This will cause him to resort to the behaviour strategies that help to get him out of situations that confuse him.

If the child is better behaved at home, as we saw above, this may be because he is a singleton and there is little pressure on him because he doesn't have to compete with siblings and may not even have to communicate at all. Added to this, he has had the attention of his parents throughout his life and therefore had many opportunities to observe their facial expressions and body language, so he may find predicting what is going on easier. But at school he hasn't had as much time to get to know the teacher's body language and mannerisms and therefore won't be able to interpret or predict so easily.

It is important to accept that different behaviours at home and at school are a reality and teachers need to work together with parents to change the situation. I have too often seen parents blamed for the behaviour of their child and yet, until now, there have been no books or advice from professionals to explain why their child is different and what they can do about it. Most books currently advise parents how to promote and deal with verbal communication but fail to address non-verbal communication.

COMPLEXITY OF GROUPS AND INTERACTIVE SPEAKING

A child with special needs which include non-verbal communication difficulties will not pick up communication skills in groups. This is because his communication development is not sufficient to make sense in all one-to-one conversational situations. Simply putting him in a group situation doesn't help as he first needs to master conversation skills in order for his social skills to have a chance of developing.

A child who is unable to process non-verbal information in one-to-one settings will only improve his skills with intervention. Non-verbal communication skills are far too complex to simply pick up in a group setting, even with support. Imagine how hard it would be to learn a new language just by joining in groups of competent speakers of that language.

The reason for this difficulty in groups is that there is a hierarchy of situations requiring more and more complex interpretational and conversational skills in order to communicate effectively. That hierarchy looks something like this:

1 One-to-one with a familiar person, ie, someone the child has known and seen daily for at least one to three months.

2 One-to-one with a less well-known person but one who uses the appropriate structure and support for his communication (see Section 12 on structure to use during the Not Just Talking intervention).

3 One-to-one with an unfamiliar person or someone who doesn't use appropriate communicative supports.

4 Small familiar group or a slightly larger group that is heavily structured.

5 Small unfamiliar group.

6 Any large group, such as playground or assembly.

The first situation is easier for children because they have seen the person on many occasions and therefore are familiar with their body language, facial expressions and tone of voice as well as their expectations. This explains why some children improve over a year at primary school – they become used to the conscious or unconscious non-verbal signals of the teacher by virtue of seeing her almost daily for a year. The child gets to know her expectations and his behaviour may improve as a result.

The child also knows the sorts of conversations to expect with parents, for example, because familiar routines such as bathing and dressing enable him to learn what is coming and help him predict what parents might be talking about. This ability to predict is central to communication, helping us among other things to know how to respond to different people (see Sections 5 and 6).

Put this child into a situation with someone he doesn't know and who doesn't use strategies for communication that would help him, and he may well resort to controlling behaviour or refuse to engage in the conversation. This is because he is unable to predict what might happen during the exchange – if he controls the conversation he can predict how it will go, or so he believes!

IMPACT OF SCHOOL

Throughout this book we have seen that school can be a serious challenge for children with poor conversational skills. Here I will discuss a few more factors likely to cause the child problems as he progresses through school.

Behaviourist approaches

At the time of writing, most of the behavioural and special needs approaches adopted in education are based on behaviourist techniques, ie, stimulus–response. As a result children can be set up to fail because these strategies teach children responses to specific signals in their environment. For instance, the child sees a symbol for 'biscuit', touches it or gives it to the teacher, and gets a biscuit. What it doesn't teach the child is how to generalise this to a range of different situations.

So children are given reward cards, targets with rewards and other stimuli. In order to gain the reward the child has to be able to replicate the behaviour. Given the same situation in the class or therapy room where he was taught this skill, he will be able to do so, but alter this slightly by putting him in a different class or a home setting and he is likely to have difficulty applying what he has learned to the new situation.

At a low level of educational ability this might not be recognised, so the expectations of those working with such children may be lower and the frequent and regular repetition of information is often standard practice. This will all help the child to generalise, but only with adult prompting. In a mainstream setting a child who has been 'told' how to behave and is given a reward card to mark his 'good' behaviour is expected to be able to repeat that behaviour in any situation. But if the child can't behave as expected because he doesn't recognise the relevant signals, he won't achieve a reward, or if he uses the behaviour inadvertently and gets a reward, he may not be able to deliberately recreate the behaviour in another setting. The problem for him is that the teacher, having seen him respond to the stimulus in one situation, might expect him to have understood and be able to apply this behaviour in a variety of situations.

Mixed-ability classes

Putting a child in a class with other children who are better communicators and expecting him to pick up conversational skills vicariously is also unrealistic. If the basic ability has not been developed, children cannot simply absorb skills from their surroundings. Children with poor non-verbal communication can only improve their skills through one-to-one intervention methods focused specifically on their individual non-verbal skills.

The same applies to trying to put children with special needs into mainstream settings without the appropriate support to develop non-verbal communication skills. Such children fare much better in settings where the academic pressure is lower and therefore puts less stress on the child to perform communicatively and academically. Once their communication skills improve to their age level, they are ready to return to mainstream school and will benefit to the full from the experience.

Effect of entering secondary school

The main issue is that a child with non-verbal communication difficulties who has nonetheless managed to survive at primary school because of the one teacher per class system is likely to find entry to secondary school a big shock.

A child might spend the whole of Year 7 trying to make friends. Here is what may happen during that year:

1   He begins by making a few friends with his peers in his tutor group because what he says fascinates them.

2   This stops working with the first tranche of peers because they realise that he doesn't show interest in what they have been doing; therefore he is unable to keep his friends.

3   He then tries to befriend another child outside the first group.

4   Soon that child is put off for the same reason.

5   The children start discussing among themselves how difficult he is to talk to.

6   Other children don't get taken in by the interesting topics on which he is particularly focused.

7   The child then has to try to make friends with children from another tutor group.

8   He quickly works his way through all the children, who find out about his poor conversational ability either from direct experience or through word of mouth.

9   Soon no one in the year wants to make friends with him.

10 By Year 8 he might be ostracised by his peers, but there is a new intake of Year 7 and he can make friends with some of these temporarily until they too find out he is a poor conversationalist.

11 He soon finds himself isolated from all of the first two years, and it is at this time, while puberty is kicking in, that things can go drastically downhill.

12 His behaviour progressively deteriorates and he is excluded from school.

Effect of different subjects

A child with poor non-verbal interpretation will tend to prefer subjects where the answers are more clear cut and do not require any discussion. So subjects such as maths or science will be of interest. Languages that no one else speaks such as Latin are also of interest because they are unusual, and because again they are relatively clear cut – you either get the words right or wrong.

But subjects such as English or History, where negotiation and discussion of possible interpretations is required, can be a severe challenge to these children and cause behaviour problems. Any child who fails to reach his educational potential should be investigated for a non-verbal communication problem.

School provision

Parents will know that there is no special school provision for mainstream children with non-verbal communication problems. The difficulty for them is that they do not have either a learning disability, mental health problems or speech and language problems.

As a result, parents often find their child excluded not only from mainstream schools but also from specialist provision. There needs to be a solution where these children can have their non-verbal communication difficulties treated in an environment that will not overload them, then as soon as their communication improves they can be moved back into a mainstream environment.

Learning disability

Boys and young teenagers with learning disabilities are particularly vulnerable as they have to learn very quickly about the complicated non-verbal messages communicated by girls and women. This is even more difficult just because they are male and find these signals harder to recognise and process. Their brain is not passing the information between the left and right cortex as swiflty as it does in women.

In learning disability, a child who has learned to talk will show the same behaviours and frustrations with communication. He may be able to talk relatively well, but if his non-verbal communication skills are lagging behind his verbal skills he will benefit from intervention to improve communication through using the Not Just Talking methods. This will enable such children to participate more effectively in their education and have better life prospects as a result.

Remember that with help a child can always promote their non-verbal skills to the same level of ability as their verbal communication. In my experience of children with moderate learning disability, verbal communication is often in advance of other skills, including non-verbal communication.

Specific learning disability

In specific learning disability, such as dyslexia, there may be an element of a communication problem that is related to non-verbal understanding. I have worked successfully with children with such difficulties, although this has not been my main caseload. My experience suggests that non-verbal interpretational difficulties are likely to be a central component of some specific learning disorders. Research could usefully be carried out in this field. Improving a child's conversational skills will have a big impact on other skill areas, including a language disability.

SOCIAL IMPACT

At the heart of socialisation is building good friendships but, as we have seen, this is a severe challenge for a child lacking essential conversational skills. He will find making friends very hard and keeping them even harder. In order to ingratiate himself into peer groups, he may start to do or say things that make them laugh or think of him as someone exciting, risky, quirky or otherwise interesting to befriend. He may also be at risk because peers may take advantage of his limited ability to predict the outcome of his actions.

Case example

One lad I met when I first started working in this way was 14 years old when I assessed him at his secondary school. I remember it well because it was a Friday afternoon. Jack had already been in trouble with the police and his teachers thought that he might be involved with either taking or selling drugs.

At assessment this 'tough' lad, who most of the teachers had labelled 'malicious' because of his evidently disruptive and aggressive behaviour in class, melted like a small child. The look in his eyes said 'At last someone knows what is wrong with me'. I arranged to start work with him the next week but over the weekend he was arrested. This precipitated a sudden move out of mainstream secondary school to a behaviour unit.

I never saw Jack again because, at that time, there was no service from the speech and language therapy department in the school he went to. I heard later in the year that he had picked up even worse behaviour and drug taking in his time at this school.

I often wonder what might have happened if I had had the opportunity to work with Jack at an earlier age – before secondary school. From all my other cases, I know that the outcome could have been very different for him.

Playing out with peers

In normal circumstances, being able to play out with friends provides the opportunity for non-verbal communication skills to be accumulated, practised and refined. But a child who has poor conversational skills will miss out on this opportunity; indeed, they may well be repeatedly falling out of friendships and running home in an upset state, and other children are less likely to call round to play. In fact, parents usually have to organise times when other children will come and play because these children don't even have sufficient skills to ask at school if another child wants to play with them.

Why do boys end up the wrong side of the law so often?

Many children – boys in particular – are vulnerable socially due to their poor interpretational skills. The really hard part for them, and for society generally, is that this can be a short and slippery road to the youth justice system. The boys I'm referring to are the ones who:

- behave inappropriately with girls and women (and sometimes men) because they can't recognise the less evident non-verbal signals that say 'Go away!' or 'Trouble!'

- are left standing at the place where they shouldn't be when the teacher or police arrive, the others having 'scarpered', leaving the boy with poor communication to deal with the consequences

- are unable to understand or answer questions adequately

- can't explain what has happened clearly enough for the police to get a reliable picture of what has actually taken place.

It is setting a person up for failure if carers allow these young people to go out into the community unaccompanied because they are not trained to understand the problems their clients will face. It is likely to be sheer good luck if such a child recognises enough of the non-verbal clues in a risky situation, is able to turn away from it and arrives home safely. And, at night or in complex situations during the daytime, he will be more vulnerable because his skills will deteriorate in these circumstances.

The drive to help people with learning disabilities live in the community is well intentioned. But even in the few years I worked in these services in the 1990s, there were episodes of vulnerable young men (mostly) being allowed out in the community on their own who, unknown to the carers, would do things at the behest of others which resulted in the police being involved. Such incidents still occur and sometimes the outcome is so serious that clients have to be incarcerated for the protection of the public.

To me this is dealing with the issue the wrong way round. Because we put people at risk of behaving inappropriately out in the community, it is our problem not the client's. But it is the client's life which is ruined as a result. The same applies in the education system, but with less dire consequences – children are blamed and excluded for behaviours that others have encouraged them to do (either knowingly or unknowingly). It is our responsibility as professionals and as a society to give these children the support they need to improve their communication skills so that they are less confused and vulnerable in the 'real' world.

Friends versus strangers

Initially a child with poor non-verbal communication will find making friends, playing with peers and keeping friends almost impossible. He will also not recognise the signals that tell him that someone is a stranger, so he may not understand that he shouldn't give that person all the information in his head about his home life, for example.

Such a child is desperate to be liked and may have found that making his peers laugh is a good way of generating what he thinks are 'friends'. If he applies these behaviours when he is older than six or seven, then his 'friends' may desert him because this behaviour will attract the wrong kind of attention from adults.

He will also do whatever his peers suggest in the hope that this will promote friendships. Of course it doesn't, and additionally he is more likely to get into trouble with teachers. As a teenager he will become even more isolated, particularly if he has become fixated with computers as a means of avoiding conversations. This can lead to depression – see below for more regarding this particular vulnerability.

IMPACT ON FAMILY

The behaviour of a child with non-verbal interpretational difficulties in the family can have a devastating impact. I have known many families where the strain of having to deal with these communication problems and the subsequent behaviours has broken up marriages and had damaging affects on siblings and other family members.

Parental expectations

In my experience, boys whose parents have divorced prefer the time spent with their fathers. This is largely because communication between men is much less convoluted than women's. Women rely more heavily on non-verbal interpretation and as a result are deemed to be better 'conversationalists'. But for such a child this means that conversation with his mother is likely to be more challenging to him than it would be with his father.

Coping strategies employed by parents

The resilience and persistence of parents never ceases to amaze me. In addition to the frustration of seeing a series of professionals who may diagnose their child as on the autistic spectrum or having autistic traits or dyspraxia or ADHD, parents have to carry on and live day-to-day with the mood swings, challenging behaviour and lack of communication of their children.

As a result of this experience, parents often learn not to interact with their child when he has 'lost it'. They send him to his room and let him come down only when he has calmed down. Often this is taken as when he is ready to say 'Sorry'.

As the boy becomes larger – I have seen a few 14-year-olds who look like front-row forwards on a rugby team – a good strategy for the mother is to have him go straight up to his room, then maybe come down for supper but go straight back up afterwards. This may help to ensure that she doesn't get hit too often, especially if she is dealing with him alone. For the child, however, this restricts his opportunities to develop the key skills because he is not observing or participating in conversations. However, this is a no-win situation – without intervention to promote conversational skills, he won't benefit from such opportunities.

Children who participate in Not Just Talking's intervention programme often show signs of improvement in school first while at home parents continue to use the strategies that have worked for them in the past. However, once the communication improves these approaches are no longer necessary:

Case example

I met Sam, a 14-year-old Asperger's boy referred to me after his exclusion from secondary school, in a pupil referral unit. The referral said something along these lines:

> *'Sioban, could you see this lad please? He is spending more time out in the playground throwing stones at the cars and at people walking through. This behaviour also results in him being sent home every day.'*

I saw Sam before Easter for assessment and he had one of the most unusual strategies for avoiding conversations that I had come across. He used a jokey or quirky response which sounded as though he was responding to what you asked but in fact was just a conversation stopper!

When asked during the assessment what made a man happy, he was unable to answer. But when prompted for more information he replied in a jokey manner, 'Well, it's not his haircut!' This was not a good interpretation as there was nothing wrong with this man's haircut, but it ended Sam's need to give information. In everyday conversations he used this technique a great deal.

Sam was very angry because he had no idea why he had been excluded from his school. On assessment, when asked what had made someone feel something, he replied, 'Why would I know that? I'm not him.'

Also, his body language was so stiff and robotic that it sounded as though he was responding to a questionnaire rather than having a conversation.

Having coped with Sam for 14 years – he was diagnosed as Asperger's at seven years – his parents were exhausted. In all that time nothing had changed. They said that they would 'never take him into a restaurant again' because his behaviour was so appalling.

The unit were at their wits' end because even with small class sizes of four or five children he refused to go into any lessons.

After six sessions given by a member of my team in the summer term, I called Sam's mum to ask how he was. Her response was 'He's still barricading himself in his room and being sent home from school!' I became a bit worried because this sounded as though there had been no change.

However, on my arrival at the unit the English teacher was on the doorstep looking excited. Sam was not only attending English lessons but participating in circle time too. When I saw him I could hardly believe the change. His humour had blossomed and now it was a part of his conversation, not something to deflect someone from communicating with him.

His body language was relaxed and it was a delight to talk to him. He was playing football when I arrived, with the peers that a few weeks earlier he had refused to talk to!

His parents, it turned out, had noticed a difference because they were taking him out to restaurants again!

That summer he was taken for his yearly assessment by the man who had known him since his diagnosis of Asperger's at seven years of age. The first thing he said was, 'What has happened to you, Sam?' This boy had not changed at all in those seven years but after six weeks of Not Just Talking intervention, his whole demeanour had been transformed.

The reason why his mother continued to react in the way she always had to Sam was because children's behaviour usually improves later at home. For her to do otherwise was too risky because if he became angered by something and started to hit out he would have done serious damage to his mother or sister. As the change in his behaviour consolidated, so she could relax and adopt a different approach to her son.

Parental concerns

Parents really struggle with these children, and because they don't get functional help from other professionals they feel very isolated. Sometimes their concerns are ignored once the assessment phase has passed and they are left to cope on their own with the children, who present increasingly difficult behaviour as they become older and larger.

I have had parents in tears because they see what Not Just Talking provides as the only help that produces a demonstrable positive change both in their child and in the problems experienced by the family. Parents also can't understand why this help was not available when they first took their child for assessment – possibly as early as three or four years of age.

Emotions and behaviour

The reason why behaviour at home can be so much worse than at school is often to do with the lack of structure in everyday living at home. Things happen in an unstructured, non-predictable manner: 'Shall we go shopping now?' or 'Quick, get your shoes and coat on, we are going to meet dad at the station'. Parents can help to ameliorate this by making clear, visual plans of what is going to happen at particular times in the day and trying not to spring changes on the child.

Children may also have difficulty understanding that if the parents are hugging another sibling they still have the same feelings for the child. I have known many cases where children with communication difficulties have taken to using knives or hurting their siblings or parents as a result of this misperception.

Problems also occur because of the child's inability to recognise that teachers have different styles of communicating. This is most noticeable at secondary school because the child will struggle with a teacher whose role is both to give pastoral care and instil discipline. It is best to keep these roles separate until the child has the skills to understand the different styles of communication.

Family rules

Children may experience a lack of clarity concerning family 'rules' because these have been generalised over a long period of time and it is assumed that everyone knows that, for instance, when they go to church they put on their best clothes or when granny comes she likes to sit in a particular chair. Parents can get over such problems by not taking for granted that the child knows the rule and always telling them the rule that is applicable in a clear manner – see the strategies to use in Section 6.

 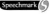

Grandparents

Grandparents can be very helpful as they have a slightly more objective eye on children than parents do. Also, they will have gained more experience of dealing with difficult situations.

But sometimes grandparents may struggle to understand the problems associated with a lack of non-verbal communication skills and as a result their expectations may be far too high. If this happens the child may come into conflict with his grandparents – or any other adult whose expectations of the child are unrealistic – and his parents will need to step in and negotiate for him.

Single parents

As we have seen, non-verbal skills are learned through modelling of conversations between two people. If there is only one parent she or he may need to make additional effort to ensure that their child has many opportunities on a daily basis to watch two people holding conversations. If there is an older sibling this is less of a problem as in normal circumstances the baby will be observing conversations between his sibling and his mother.

Preparing to return to school after holiday

A difficult time for children with poor interpretation and prediction skills is the transfer from home to school, particularly at the end of a holiday. This is magnified if the child is transferring between schools, say from infant to junior or junior to secondary.

The child will use deflection or distraction techniques to avoid situations where this is spoken about, and the parents' only recourse will be to:

- create a visual timetable containing all the good things that will happen before the date of returning to school

- have photos available of his new class teacher and his classmates

- make daily reference to these visual clues in the build-up to the return to school

- explain carefully when buying shoes and clothes that these are for school purposes.

What clothes communicate

In Section 2 we saw how important clothes are for helping us to understand what is going on in situations. Also, it is important that children have a positive self-image of themselves as a child, so dressing a young child in 'grown-up' clothes removes a key opportunity for him to be a child and have childlike experiences.

For girls it is more complex. Her expectations and those of people she encounters are raised when a girl of six, seven or eight is dressed like a teenager because the non-verbal signals are out of sync with her age. As Sue Palmer (2006) agrees, children need to grow up slowly, and it takes all their life-experiences as children through to the end of their teenage years to accumulate the necessary skills. If we dress children as adults, it catapults them into adult life before their time, placing additional strain on their communication.

LANGUAGE PROBLEMS

The most common language difficulty identified with conventional Speech and Language assessments is that the child has a mismatch between his skills of comprehension and expression. Whereas such children are likely to have poor articulation, vocabulary or grammar and low levels of verbal understanding, children with non-verbal communication problems often exhibit excellent verbal language skills and only a relatively minor problem with their language comprehension.

Language comprehension

The ability to understand what is being said to you is not simply based on whether or not you understand the words used and have good auditory discrimination and sequencing skills. You can be good at all these skill areas but still have problems in understanding what is being said to you.

So a child who is unable to use the 60–90 per cent of non-verbal clues to help him interpret the message will have a profile which shows lower than expected verbal understanding, especially when looked at alongside his verbal language use, which is likely to be very good.

He may also demonstrate auditory memory problems, which are not usually due to a particular difficulty with auditory memory, but because he is unable to remember all the words spoken to him in an utterance. If he is processing the non-verbal information correctly, his auditory memory will only be required to focus on the information-carrying words. This also applies to auditory sequencing skills.

In my experience, both comprehension of language and auditory memory problems improve when the child has benefited from the Not Just Talking intervention and his interpretational skills have developed.

Use of spoken language

Problems with either grammar or vocabulary should improve automatically as a by-product of the child's improved participation in conversations – he is learning how to construct sentences by listening more carefully to what is said to him. Really complex difficulties will require more direct help, but again this will be easier because the child is better equipped to participate.

Articulation

I have found that children of six years plus who still have articulation difficulties –

usually lisps and lateral /s/ but sometimes more complex problems – respond quickly and well to the usual speech and language therapy techniques for working on these difficulties once their conversational skills are improving. I also think that if a child reaches this age without having benefited from intervention at an earlier age, then it would be very remiss not to improve these residual articulatory problems.

It is a matter of concern that, with the reduction in speech and language therapy provision in the UK since the 1990s, children over school entry age are unlikely to receive intervention. In an attempt to make best use of limited resources, speech and language therapists concentrate on the early years. If speech, language and communication services in all children's services adopted the methods advocated here, they could then work effectively and in a time-limited fashion with children under and over the age of seven.

Vocabulary

Usually with non-verbal communication difficulties, vocabulary is not a problem with regard to the child's area of special interest; however, there is often a paucity of vocabulary relating to everyday activities. Not Just Talking intervention techniques enable a child to begin to experience those everyday activities in such a way as to acquire the vocabulary effectively. As a result his vocabulary should develop normally. However, if he is still struggling to relate semantic categories, normal speech and language therapy techniques will work more effectively as a result of his improved understanding of the conversational process.

Grammar

A common grammatical problem that can persist after a child with a language disorder reaches the age where his conversational difficulties are causing more problems than his language difficulties is the use of pronouns and personal pronouns. I have worked with quite a few children who enter the programme with problems with 'he' and 'she' and 'his' and 'hers', but by simply asking the question when they provide the wrong pronoun for example 'Is it a boy?', they usually learn to self-correct, because of the improvement in their conversation skills.

Working on language

Working on a child's language is detrimental if his non-verbal communication skills are functioning at a lower level. It is still possible to improve a child's language skills in these circumstances, but this will most likely lead to an increased separation between language and non-verbal skills. If the non-verbal skills are worked on and not the language, any residual language problems should be overcome by increasingly effective participation in conversations.

The non-verbal child

A child who fails to learn to talk comes under one or more of the following categories:

• His non-verbal skills have not reached the point at which spoken language develops. In normal development this is at any time between 12 and 36 months. So a child with a learning disability might not reach this stage, without help, before the age of 10 years or more, depending on the severity of the learning disability. Whatever the case, trying to teach him to talk before this point is reached is not just a waste of your time but a waste of precious time for the child's development potential.

• He may have a specific language disorder.

• He might have an articulatory dyspraxia. This means that, despite being able to eat and drink and so move his organs of articulation spontaneously, the moment he tries to make the tongue or lips or palate do a volitional act , say, closing for a plosive sound such as /p/, he cannot move his articulators at all or can do so only partially. I once worked with a child who was totally unable to use his articulators for communicative purposes. I recently caught up with him at the age of 15 and he is still non-verbal but communicates through his iPod, which has a voice communicator that speaks his messages.

DEVELOPMENTAL DISORDERS

Usually, if a child is diagnosed with a disorder in his development there is an element of communication impairment. Here I will discuss some particular problems associated with these disorders.

Autistic spectrum

In this section I will cover children diagnosed with autism and Asperger's syndrome. An autistic diagnosis is likely to have accompanying learning disability and the child may also be non-verbal. However an Asperger's diagnosis has good verbal language skills and generally a higher level of IQ.

Problems with diagnosis

Because research is so focused on the development of verbal communication skills and thought, generally it is felt that it is not appropriate to make a diagnosis of autism before the child is about three or four, unless the signs are quite obvious, and sometimes this diagnosis is not made until much later. With more research into non-verbal elements of communication, it would be easier to see which babies are at risk of developing autistic spectrum behaviours and then do something that is likely to halt progress on this route.

A baby who is unable to develop in all areas described in Section 4 may be on the autistic spectrum. However, if these essential skills are promoted, and the temptation to get the baby to 'talk' is resisted, the child may well reveal themselves to be less autistic than was first thought. In my experience, assessing young babies and starting early intervention ensures that children grow up with a better chance of communicating effectively. This applies to all babies, including those likely to be autistic.

Another problem I see with diagnosis is that time and again children who behave differently at home and in school are diagnosed on the autistic spectrum. In my speech and language therapy training, one of the tenets that I took as gospel was that autism is a pervasive disorder. At a basic level this means that if you are autistic, you are autistic in all situations. It is not possible to be autistic at school but not at home and vice versa. So when children can communicate in one situation but not another, a diagnosis of autism should not be made.

I have had many experiences where parents are confused because teachers are telling them that their child is an 'angel' in school and at home he is a huge challenge. These parents can't understand why their child can function so well at school but the minute he arrives home he becomes aggressive and hurtful.

Another real difficulty with diagnosis currently faced by psychologists and other professionals is that their training does not include the development of non-verbal aspects of communication discussed in this book. So it is the communication difficulty which really stands out when they see a child. These children arrive with all the symptoms of non-verbal communication disorders. For example, they:

- don't look at the other person when speaking

- can't keep still

- have histories of significant behavioural and social difficulties

- can't talk about what the assessor wants them to

- have other unusual communicative habits

- don't have theory of mind.

But because the triad of impairments (see below) says that these behaviours are not related to communication, it is easy to misdiagnose a child.

Communication is central to autism. The symptoms exhibited by some children on the autistic spectrum are behaviours adopted to deal with their communication difficulty. And the fact that in one situation they can behave in a manner people see as 'normal' can be explained by the following reasons and is not anything to do with the skills or attitudes of parents:

1 The child is holding himself tight at school in order not to display the behaviours that he knows upset his parents but is unable to do anything about.

2 He is able to process the non-verbal information at school because school has slightly more structure than home life so he is able to understand rules and signals more easily.

3   At home he is competing for his parent's attention with his siblings, whereas at school there is a more structured approach to apportioning the teacher's attention. There will be an orderly queue for the teacher's attention, while at home it is the survival of the fittest.

4   As a consequence of 'scripts' that are used in school, he quickly picks up what to say or do at a signal from the teacher, for instance, at registration or when the teacher claps her hands all the class stand still and listen.

5   At school he finds talking to the adults much easier and tends to seek them out in situations where he is less likely to be interrupted by his peers, such as playground supervision.

6   There is a predictability at school and often a bell to signal the end of class and start of playtime. At home, life can be spontaneous and unpredictable.

Taking all these factors into account, and recognising that in some situations the child is able to make sense of what is going on and to communicate effectively, suggests to me he is not on the autistic spectrum. No child who is able to communicate relatively well one-to-one with a familiar adult should be viewed as showing autistic-like behaviours.

The triad of impairments

The triad of impairments that make up an autistic diagnosis are:

1   communication impairment

2   social impairment

3   lack of imagination – leading to obsessive behaviours.

Obviously, the first impairment relates to communication but social impairment is also communication based. Without conversational skills we are unable to socialise and those on the autistic spectrum have a fundamental difficulty either at a verbal or a non-verbal level in using conversations to communicate.

Finally, the child's confidence around a favoured topic and his inability to converse on topics generated by others could make him appear to have a lack of imagination. So this is also communication based. As it is possible to improve the conversational skills of all verbal children through intervention, all three areas of the triad will improve.

Autism

In autism, as Leo Kanner originally described in 1943, there is likely to be a lack of language to use for communicative purposes combined with an inability to relate to people. This is associated with a real desire to avoid change by keeping everything the same. So a child will appear obsessed with controlling his environment, maintaining everything in a state of sameness. Because of the severity of their communication difficulties, autistic children may never achieve their educational potential.

Using the Not Just Talking assessment techniques, it is possible to identify babies soon after birth who are at risk of developing problems associated with the autistic spectrum. If this is achieved, a programme can be devised to promote the development of essential communication skills. This will improve the child's ability to relate to people and he should go on to cope with change. In autism it might just take a longer period of time.

I have also worked successfully with older children with severe autism, even teenagers, and in periods of about a year they have developed skills such as an interest in faces and the ability to choose with meaning. If the work started under the age of six months, the task should be a great deal easier and more effective.

Asperger's syndrome

Children with Asperger's syndrome often have a history of learning to talk early, sometimes before one year. This is also an indicator for non-verbal problems. If a child learns to talk too early then he won't have sufficient time to develop the essential non-verbal communication that underpins his speech. The talking is then promoted by everyone who is in contact with the child and the language skills quickly outstrip the non-verbal communication skills. Over time the gap between the two just gets larger.

Children I have worked with who have been diagnosed as Asperger's owing to their lack of imagination are usually able to talk imaginatively about their topic of interest. In my view, the symptoms of lack of imagination are often based on the fact that the child is obsessed with certain topics of conversation. This is a result of his being unable to talk about other topics. This obsession with topics disappears after intervention and all children demonstrate an ability to talk about most topics in their daily life.

Children also prefer to talk about what they know because this gives them confidence and, in their eyes, the subject is of interest to others. This may be a good thing up to the age of about six, but after that their topic dominance becomes an impairment to socialisation. Socialisation is totally dependent on conversational skills.

So you can see that all three impairments are interlinked by communication. You can't change the elements of autism, but if a child's non-verbal communication skills are improved, he will communicate better as long as he has opportunities to develop experiential skills. As a result of being able to hold conversations in all situations, some children who have been diagnosed as having Asperger's syndrome cease to demonstrate the behaviours that gave rise to their diagnosis. They can then go on to achieve their potential academically, socially and emotionally as well.

So my recommendation is, that before a lifelong diagnosis of autism or Asperger's is made, a child is given the benefit of assessment of their non-verbal communication skills to ascertain whether he just has a major communication problem and in fact is not on the autistic spectrum.

Theory of mind

Currently, theory of mind is seen as central to the diagnosis of Asperger's syndrome. What you will see here is that this is also a communication skill that is remediable, whether or not the child has another diagnosis such as Asperger's or autism.

Alan Leslie first brought the idea of 'theory of mind' to the fore in 1985 while researching into autistic impairments, in a paper published in the American Psychological Association journal, Psychological Review. He reports that children start developing the ability to pretend during the second year of life and this is dependent on the skill of being able to represent objects and situations. He sees theory of mind as a consequence of 'pretending' skills which, in my opinion, develop on the foundation of non-verbal skills referred to in this book.

What does it mean?

'Theory of mind' relates to the ability to put oneself into another's shoes and see the world from a perspective other than one's own. This is a fundamental communication skill because, as we have already seen, understanding what another person is thinking enables us to know what to say to them since we can predict what they need to know and how they might react.

Simon Baren-Cohen (2004) says that 'theory of mind' or 'mind reading' are part of cognitive empathy (a term employed by the pioneering child psychologist Jean Piaget), and that this is combined with an affective component which is bound up in the communication because it determines 'an observer's appropriate emotional response to another person's emotional state'.

Children diagnosed with autism do not have this skill, in my view because they have missed out on the early communication skills which are developed before the age of one or two. I suggest that it is possible to diagnose much earlier a child who is susceptible to being on the autistic spectrum by ascertaining whether the child:

- has an interest in faces

- can anticipate

- is starting to take turns while feeding

- has self- and other awareness

- is able to deal with change.

Any child unable to do any of these things can be encouraged to do so by using the suggestions in Not Just Talking: Helping Your Baby Communicate – From Day One (Boyce, 2009). Children who don't pick up these skills easily and need individual support of more than three months could then be deemed to be on the autistic spectrum. But even this group would improve at this early age if the skills were promoted with consistency for as long as it took for the child to acquire them.

Implications for communication

Because he is unable to put himself in the shoes of another person and know what they might be feeling or thinking, a child without theory of mind will not know what to say to people. He will assume that his thoughts and those of others are the same and therefore that he has no need to communicate. Our drive to communicate happens when we know that what is in our brain is different from someone else's.

The reason why the Not Just Talking intervention programme is so successful in producing theory of mind in children is because the child learns how to recognise what people are feeling from their body language and facial expressions, and the therapy relates this improved understanding to what might happen and what the child might say in response to different emotional states.

Situational understanding

Remember that autism will cause a problem with situational understanding, but with more serious consequences than for a mainstream child who has good skills in other areas. But as with the latter group of children, learning to focus on non-verbal signals pertaining to different situations will help communication.

I have a theory as to why some children, known as 'savants', have exceptional skills in one particular area. The child may be able to:

- draw complex buildings or landscapes with photographic precision

- play amazing music without having been taught to play

- recite all the prime numbers to infinity.

If you think of the brain as a computer, then the amount of 'RAM' (random access memory) taken up constantly by processing non-verbal (visual, aural, contextual) information is phenomenal. However, if you are unable to process this information, imagine how much free brain capacity that would give you. So children with non-verbal communication difficulties lack the wealth of information that we store daily for the experiential component of non-verbal communication and this enables them to focus on one particular area.

My interpretation of these 'savants' is that their topic interest fills their lives, because it gives confidence and recognition from society. It tends also to keep those awkward conversations at bay because people only want to talk about your amazing talent. But what happens when a child does not have this level of skill and may in fact have a learning disability or when a 'savant' has to communicate outside his topic of interest? He will take on board all the non-verbal information available in the form of 'raw data', which will lead to severe confusion and a great desire to get out of the situation that is causing it. And he will become anxious and stressed as a result.

Generalisation from situation to situation

In autism (and other aspects of learning disability) one of the biggest problems educationally is the lack of an ability to generalise. This means that the child cannot transfer a skill or information learned in one situation to another – a big impediment to learning and one which affects everything from their communication development to educational progress and socialisation.

However, working with the Not Just Talking intervention programme for the past 15 years has shown that one of the most satisfying outcomes is that a child learns to generalise quickly and easily. He is taught how to recognise the signals in a situation that provide a guide to what to say and do; they are identified and reinforced in the next situation or situations; and he learns to apply this information to tell him what to say and do in each new set of circumstances. Having had very negative experiences of communicating in different situations, he is soon able to generalise and this gives him confidence and improves his self-esteem.

Use of non-verbal communication

Children on the autistic spectrum usually have disordered development of their expressive non-verbal communication skills, just as their language is likely to be disordered. So look for signs of odd body language which might be completely eccentric or lacking for normal day-to-day conversations, or intonation patterns that are flat and monotonous or always exaggerated. These aspects of communication will improve, but probably not automatically as they would for children who are not on the autistic spectrum. The child is likely to require direct work on use of body language and intonation patterns. But this should only be implemented when his conversational skills are good.

Speech and language problems

Improvement in residual language problems can be achieved much more easily once the child's conversational skills improve. In fact, during the intervention I have found it easy to make changes in all these areas, including residual problems such as lateral /s/ or /r/, and grammatical features such as subject–verb concordance and personal pronoun use.

Facial interest

As most researchers agree, a lack of facial interest is one of the major indicators of autism. However, the diagnosis should not be predicated on this feature alone. People often say that a child is 'not interested' in looking at faces. No adult should ever assume that a child under the age of six or seven years, and later if there is a learning disability, is 'choosing' not to look at them. Children do not have the skill to know why looking at people is so important communicatively and if they are not taught to do this through modelling or more direct work on this skill, then the child won't develop this necessary understanding.

So once more a diagnosis should not be made until the child has benefited from intervention focused on fostering an interest in faces. In my experience, young children with Asperger's or autistic tendencies can be helped to develop a normal interest in reading faces in a short time. Once the child appreciates the benefit of looking at faces, he will want to do so because it helps him communicate more easily. Interest in facial expressions can be promoted in severe cases of learning disability and autism if every subject taught has this target as its basis.

Attention deficit hyperactivity disorder

As I hope is clear, keeping still is one of the most important aspects of learning how to communicate and going on to hold effective conversations. All that I want to say here is that, because ADHD has at its centre an inability to keep still, then such children are going to have some degree of non-verbal communication difficulty.

As with any child who is unable to keep still on entry to the Not Just Talking intervention programme, giving some attention to helping them recognise the benefit to communication of being still will eradicate the wriggling. Every child I have worked with has stopped fidgeting, wriggling or jumping up and down.

Elective/selective mutes

The basis of mutism is that the child decides when and when not to talk. The children that I treat do this too. So it appears to me that a child who elects not to talk in certain situations is likely to have an interpretational difficulty which should respond to the Not Just Talking intervention. Again, research is needed to clarify this.

Stammers

Stammering, looked at from the non-verbal perspective and in particular with regard to the strategies adopted by children to deal with their difficulty in understanding what is said to them, also looks like a delaying tactic. It allows the stammerer time to process what is being said and what he is trying to say. It also is a fairly good method of controlling conversations – again, akin to what children with poor non-verbal communication skills want to do.

Genetic factors

For years research was carried out to find a genetic connection between generations in families with autistic children or antecedents. When I investigated this during the first year of an EdD, I found that what the researchers were looking for was evidence of autism. However, when I read the research findings with my expertise I could see clear evidence of a non-verbal communication problem in the different generations. Because the researchers couldn't find autism in each generation they concluded that there was no link. It took many years to eventually find a link, which might have been made sooner had the focus been on non-verbal communication.

Vaccinations

There has been a great deal of controversy over the combined mumps, measles and rubella (MMR) vaccination. Here are just a few questions about its introduction in the late 1980s.

- This introduction occurred at a time when the number of children with non-verbal communication difficulties increased exponentially. At this time an educational psychologist said to me about the growth in behaviour problems in schools, 'What is going on, Sioban? Is there something in the water?'

- Research has always looked for a link between autism and the vaccine but never found it. Again, I suspect that a link might have been identified if the children were assessed for non-verbal communication difficulties rather than autism.

- This is not the single cause, but may be one of the factors combining to create such a massive increase in non-verbal communication difficulties.

Vulnerabilities

Children with poor non-verbal communication skills are very vulnerable, particularly with regard to 'stranger danger'. Young children under three are more likely to go happily with people who are kind and appear to know them because their ability to interpret and predict is insufficiently advanced. Older children whose skills are at a level commensurate with a three-year-old or younger will exhibit the same kind of behaviour.

Banter

Children and adults – particularly those cared for by staff in homes – struggle to keep up with conversations. Banter is an advanced form of conversation, often employing sarcasm, irony or coded messages, and should not be used with teenagers in the expectation that they will understand what is being said or learn to join in. Children with these non-verbal communication difficulties won't recognise all the nuances in banter for what they are and will end up confused and anxious as a result.

I have often witnessed this happening in care homes for youngsters. Staff members have conversations between themselves in the presence of the children and the outcome is either that the children just don't understand what is being said and so feel left out of the conversation, or they pick up phrases that they apply inappropriately in other situations.

Bullying

These children are vulnerable to being seen as a bully – because they don't pick up the clues telling them when to stop a conversation because it is hurting another person. Also conversationally they say the wrong things at the wrong time, which can make others think they are being rude, aggressive or bullying.

Or they can be vulnerable to being bullied themselves. This is because they are unable to be assertive and feel incapable of keeping up with the conversation. This undermines their confidence, which in turn makes them more vulnerable to bullying.

Adults should be aware of this vulnerability and the fact that it applies to both ends of the bullying spectrum. Conversational skills should be assessed before assuming that the child is choosing to act as a bully.

Alcohol and drugs

A child with poor non-verbal communication wants to be liked but struggles to make friends, so when offered alcohol or drugs he is likely to participate because:

1 he wants to be accepted into the friendship group

2   he doesn't understand the consequences of either alcohol or drug taking.

He finds saying 'no' more difficult as he feels that people will not like him if he does so and therefore he may well move on quickly to harder substance abuse.

Depression and suicide

A child who is unable to understand the change in his emotions during adolescence and certainly not the change in the feelings communicated by others will find this time especially challenging. Remember that he will have few friends as a result of his communication difficulty and even if he did have friends he would not be able to share his experiences with them because his conversational skills would not permit it. This can quickly lead to depression and may even spiral downwards to suicide if not recognised and treated.

Many of the teenage children referred to Not Just Talking were depressed at the start of intervention to the extent that some might have considered suicide. However, improving their communication skills improved their feelings and because they were able to engage with their peers more meaningfully and make some friends their depression lifted. Excellent film evidence on the Not Just Talking website (www.notjusttalking.co.uk) shows a very depressed 14-year-old, who worried his mother a great deal, blooming into a confident, outgoing 19-year-old. This transition actually occurred within a year of starting the intervention.

Vulnerability to crime

The effect of being unable to predict the consequences of his actions can very quickly put a child on the slippery slope to committing crime and ending up in the prison service. Once in prison, he will be vulnerable to further deterioration in his behaviour because he is likely to reflect and adopt the very high levels of anger and frustration communicated by those around him. People with poor non-verbal interpretation do not notice more moderate levels of feelings so appear to ignore them, but bold high-level feelings will be picked up and used – appropriately or inappropriately.

Consider a young man released on parole from an institution in which he had been placed because of inappropriate behaviour with a woman he didn't know when he left secondary school.

This man had a severe communication problem which left him able to talk but severely lacking in non-verbal communication skills. On parole he was placed in the community in a secure unit. But in the unit the staff assumed that his communication was much better than in fact it was. Gradually they gave him opportunities, as they saw it, to develop socialisation skills – by allowing him out, very occasionally, on his own.

However, on one occasion he saw a young woman and followed her and said or did something to really upset her. He was then sent back to the institution with no prospect of ever coming out again.

The problem was that the service he was released into did not understand that he didn't have the skills to know what behaviour was appropriate in many situations, including those involving women. So letting him out in the hope that he would pick up the skills was in fact setting him up for failure. He was simply not equipped to learn from observing other people, and even if he had been, those useful learning situations occur less frequently once you are an adult. Most development of these skills happens in the teenage years and during this time he was in a single-sex institution.

So we really need to be careful not to make assumptions about the behaviour of people and children who have never had the opportunity to develop these essential skills. I am now going to look at a particular case where something similar may have happened.

The James Bulger murder

I wish to make no excuses for the awful crime committed by Jon Venables and Robert Thompson in 1993, but it is interesting to speculate what might have been revealed if those professionals who were responsible for them earlier in their lives had assessed their non-verbal communication skills.

These are the case histories of the two boys gained from Times Online (Booth, 2010):

- Venables was described as having tantrums after his parents separated when he was four – presumably this had been on the cards for a while, and as the years before entry to school are crucial for the development of non-verbal understanding, he would have been at risk.

- There was a mismatch at school between performance and potential (key signs of poor non-verbal communication skills), along with not following instructions.

- His behaviour deteriorated and he became physically more aggressive (a child with poor interpretation will become increasingly confused and resort to aggressive behaviour to get himself out of the conversation).

- He reported bullying – children with poor non-verbal skills are very vulnerable to either being bullied or being seen as bullies.

- His mother reported a different child at home – loving and caring but hyperactive.

- He was jealous of attention towards his siblings from his mother.

- He had to change school because of physical aggression to another child – he would not have been able to cope with banter.

- When he changed school he met Thompson, who had been kept down a year because he was a 'misfit'.

- The firm control of a male teacher meant that Venables coped well in class – this is understandable because he would have been consistent, firm and clear.

- But Venables couldn't cope in the playground – another indicator of non-verbal communication difficulties.

- His next teacher felt that Thompson was more manipulative and led Venables into trouble in school, including truanting and shoplifting – children with non-verbal difficulties often are drawn to other children who may also have a problem but one which manifests itself in a slightly different way.

- Thompson was the fifth child of parents who quarrelled a lot when he was young.

- There were times when his father hit his mother.

- In a family who only use one or two styles of communication, a child will find it hard to pick up different ways of doing things.

- When he was six, his parents separated and his father had no contact with the children.

- His older siblings began truanting and were involved in petty crime – they would have been another poor model for Thompson.

- He watch adult-rated videos – for any child this is not helpful but for a child who is already having trouble with processing non-verbal information and probably cannot tell the difference between reality and fiction, watching these types of films would be most detrimental – see below for more on this.

So as a result of failing to develop sufficient communication skills these two boys were led astray by a series of events that neither of them would have been wholly responsible for. Their predictive skills would have been extremely low and it is unlikely that they fully anticipated the consequences of what they were doing. However, everyone else assumed that they had the skills to understand what they had done.

Both boys were vulnerable for different reasons and as a result of not being able to process non-verbal information they ended up truanting from school. At the age of two their victim, James Bulger, would not have developed the non-verbal communication skills to understand the implications of leaving his mum and going with the boys.

An educational psychology assessment of Venables appeared only to be able to describe how he behaved rather than identify what might be causing his problems.

The fact that the boys told others they met along the way to the railway line stories about James being their brother or that he was lost and they were taking him to the police station is seen as evidence that they knew what they were doing. Children who watch adult films about similar situations – perhaps involving the police – will learn the 'right' things to say as a parrot would; someone asks the question in the right way and they will know the answer that is required. This does not guarantee that they fully understand what they are saying or its consequences.

As I say, I am not an apologist for the boys, nor do I wish to appear alarmist. This was an exceptionally rare and extreme case. However, it gives a possible indication of the value of being able to detect and treat non-verbal communication problems at an early age. There are many cases of people in prison now who arrived there because they were vulnerable – they were unable to interpret situations correctly or choose the appropriate behaviour for the situation.

Television/screens

A child who finds conversations difficult and confusing will choose to interact with screens because they don't talk back or ask awkward questions. So a behaviour such as watching TV or playing on the computer is an excellent way to avoid participating in conversations.

However, as we saw in the case history of Raymond above, watching screens does not mean that you are able to understand what is being shown. So children may become exceedingly worried about subjects that they have not really understood, such as violence or pornography. Or they might become dulled to the implications of these particular subjects.

Remember that children with poor non-verbal understanding will not know reality from fantasy and may apply behaviours they see which could put them at serious risk – such as superheroes who jump off the top of buildings. They may also be likely to hit out at people and be surprised at them getting hurt.

CONCLUSION

This section has covered the problems that you will come across in children who have non-verbal communication skill difficulties, but not all children will have a full complement of these problems. Some will have very good skills in some of the areas discussed masking an underlying weakness in another area or areas which will impact on the child – particularly on entry to secondary school if not before. By developing the missing skills, intervention can reduce or remove the problems described here.

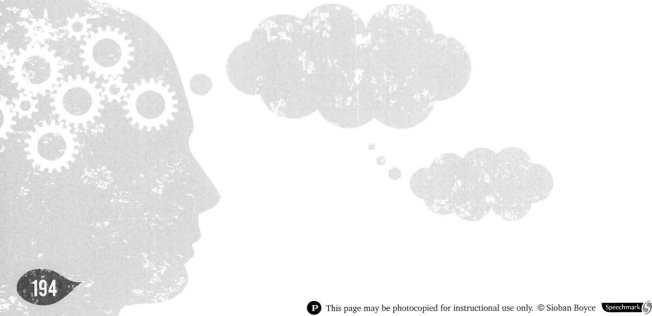

PREVENTION

10

This is a parent-based solution that can be used to support parents in promoting these essential non-verbal communication skills. This section will give an outline of what you can do to help parents. Parents who promote these skills will avoid the consequences of having a child who develops social, emotional and behavioural difficulties and is unable to benefit from her education.

■ HOW CAN NON-VERBAL COMMUNICATION PROBLEMS BE PREVENTED?

There is a relatively small window in which it is possible for parents to promote the acquisition of non-verbal skills in their children. The earlier they begin the better. Once the child starts talking, it may be far harder to prevent the longer-term problems outlined in this book just by following the recommendations in this section.

Once a child starts talking well, her complex language will make preventative work very hard and she is more than likely to respond only to the Not Just Talking intervention programme. So parents could start using these techniques from the first day until about four or five years of age.

Older children with a learning disability

Children who fail to learn to talk because of a learning disability will also benefit from these techniques until the time they start talking. This might be before or after 10 years of age but the skills required will be the same – it will just take longer to establish them.

Staff in a secondary school for severe learning disability may need to focus on promoting interest in faces for as much as a year before a child develops this skill. The main thing is not to give up. It is also possible to achieve prediction and anticipation through the persistent use of nursery rhymes, for instance. It is also appropriate to use these with older children who are functioning at a pre-three-year-old level with regard to their non-verbal communication development.

Prevention of communication problems in associated disorders

It is possible to identify children who are at risk of autistic spectrum diagnosis and using the Not Just Talking prevention techniques will ensure that these children are better able to communicate and live lives that are more fulfilled as a result. There is more about this in Sections 11 and 12.

CONCLUSION

In Section 13 you will find out more about prevention because it is so much easier to prevent these non-verbal communication difficulties than to live with the consequences later in the child's life. Parents can be encouraged to implement some simple and intuitive methods of helping their baby to develop these essential communication skills and give them a sure foundation that will serve her for the rest of her life.

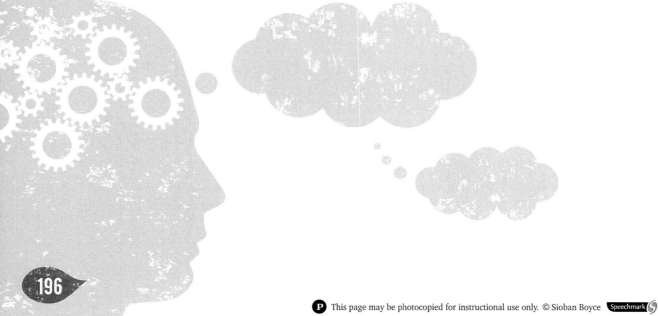

'SHINING THROUGH: THE NOT JUST TALKING APPROACHES'

ASSESSMENT

11

The assessment I devised to identify a lack of non-verbal interpretational skills could easily be developed into a screening tool for pre-school children to eliminate problems in all areas of communication. This section will demonstrate how this is possible and why the assessment is so effective.

I will describe the Not Just Talking Assessment in outline. The full programme may only be used by those who are trained in assessment techniques. It is anticipated that the full NJT assessment programme will be published in 2012.

The full assessment has been devised using current resources available in Colorcards© (Speechmark Publishing Ltd). These work adequately, but because they have not been specifically designed for the needs of this assessment they are not ideal. It is hoped that Speechmark will publish this assessment in the next few years. The assessment can only be done by those people who have a professional qualification during which they have undergone assessment training, such as psychologists, specialist teachers and health professionals. A screening method to help identify interpretational problems is available for others such as class teachers and learning support assistants. This will be part of the Not Just Talking Intervention Pack.

WHY IS A NEW ASSESSMENT NEEDED?

Current standardised language assessments focus on identifying developmental norms of language – comprehension and expression. These assessments establish the child's language level and plan a programme based on achieving 'normal language' capability.

The children I am talking about, who are good at the verbal expressive language element of these assessments, are often discharged from speech and language therapy services as a result of scoring well on verbal skills. The discharged children are then left to fend for themselves with the consequences already covered elsewhere in this book. Often these were the children who ended up being referred to Not Just Talking.

Because language comprehension tests are not structured in the manner of the Not Just Talking assessment, they do not, in my opinion, give a valid result. How can you say that a child doesn't understand something if, due to an information-giving problem unrelated to comprehension, they tell you something different from what you have asked? The question then becomes: 'Does the child understand what is asked but simply cannot answer, or is he choosing not to answer?'

To compound the problem, his verbal comprehension will be reduced automatically because he is listening to every word (as he is not able to access the 60–90 per cent of non-verbal information available to him), and as all professionals know, we cannot remember all the words when someone is speaking at 120 words per minute. Alternatively, owing to the confusion caused by his non-verbal interpretational problems, he may just not answer at all.

Who would you use this assessment for?

The assessment is only used with children who have good expressive language skills. They do not need to be perfect, but if the child has poor verbal communication, limited to one- or two-word utterances when talking about his preferred topics, then see the section below on assessment for non-verbal children.

What are the symptoms of a child with non-verbal communication problems?

This is what you should look for if you are concerned about a child's communication either before he starts school or on entry to school. If a child shows signs of any or some of these behaviours, you should question whether their non-verbal communication skills are adequately developed. Failure to address these will lead to problems – perhaps not until KS2 or secondary school or even only at home – but they will occur.

Signs from what he says

These will include:

- mainly good verbal expression skills – no problems with articulation, grammar or vocabulary (the latter for preferred topics)

- limited vocabulary when talking about what someone else wants to talk about

- tends to talk exclusively about his own favourite topics

- language skills diminish as soon as he becomes anxious about giving information that others request

- difficulty answering supplementary questions

- wants to dominate the conversation all the time

- doesn't give way to others

- won't wait for his turn to talk

- may appear to bully others

- inappropriate content, such as asking a vicar what colour knickers his wife wears

- talks in a way that assumes you have knowledge of or experience of situations you obviously do not, for example, assumes you were out in the playground watching or participating in his play.

Signs from his listener skills

He may do any or all of these:

- not look at the speaker

- fidget

- not answer questions adequately or at all

- give irrelevant information

- interrupt inappropriately

- not appreciate that what someone is saying to the group applies to him

- not give non-verbal feedback to what he hears.

Non-verbal communication signs

These include:

- body direction will not allow him to look at people when talking to them

- may not look at people sufficiently when talking to them, ie, looks away too quickly and fails to look back, or only looks when he has finished speaking

- doesn't look at people enough as a listener or just doesn't look at all

- lack of facial expression

- expression changes rarely or not at all

- limited or no use of body language

- exaggerated use of body language.

Signs from his behaviour

He may display some or all of the following:

- temper tantrums when he doesn't get his own way

- sudden inexplicable eruption of excessive anger

- physical or verbal aggression

- total withdrawal from communication

- flight

- preference to be on his own

- lack of friends

- continuing to do something despite being told repeatedly not to

- no awareness of the impact of what he says or does.

Any combination of these symptoms should prompt you to query his non-verbal skills and put him forward for assessment.

THE NOT JUST TALKING ASSESSMENT

This new assessment was devised to be efficient and cost-effective for parents, who initially were the largest purchasers of Not Just Talking's services. Within half an hour, at the most, it gives a complete overview of language development as well as all the information needed regarding the child's non-verbal communication skills.

It comprises four sections:

1 Free conversation – can the child give good information that meets the needs of his listener?

2 Emotion pictures – can the child give the information required to make full sense of the basic emotions of happy, sad and angry?

3 What's Wrong pictures – a bit of light relief which often identifies significant difficulties with prediction or even picking up what is wrong.

4 Story sequence – a five-card sequence where the child has to be able to predict from the body language of more than one person and make good sense of what is going on.

Children fall into two main camps: either they take the full half-hour (or more for an inexperienced assessor) or the assessment might only last for 15 minutes or less. Either situation will give all the information necessary to assess the problems of the child because:

- if the child talks far too much the assessment will take half an hour or more. This will demonstrate that he has a problem knowing how much information to give or whether or not the listener is interested in his information

- if the child can't give information (the assessment is abandoned if the child shows serious signs of being unable to provide the information) you will know the child has a major information-giving problem and can plan intervention based on the level of his breakdown.

Quite often the children are able to give information to a certain level in response to the first card but then things can rapidly go downhill. The usual point to abandon the assessment is after the first or second card in the sequence, towards the end of the assessment. This sequence puts a very high load on the child's non-verbal processing skills and if the assessor doesn't pick up these signals, the child is likely to resort to his avoidance behaviours.

In 15 years of assessing and working with children with significant behaviour problems I have never been hurt or attacked. This is because I never push them beyond their capacity to process information.

Video evidence

The session is recorded on video – this is vital because from the first day of assessment the child begins to change. This is due to the following factors:

1 The child usually becomes aware that the assessor knows the basis of his communication problem and that she will be able to do something to help him.

2 After the assessment, the results are immediately shared with parents and school personnel who have day-to-day interactions with the child.

3 This means that their viewpoint changes and they start to understand his confusion, enabling them to provide appropriate support and encouragement.

4 The basic strategies that are given at this stage work for the child and produce a more positive outcome for communication for everyone concerned.

Non-verbal interpretation skills

The main focus of the assessment is to discover whether the child is able to interpret appropriately all the necessary non-verbal information to make best sense of the verbal language he hears. As we will see later in this section, this includes getting an idea about his information-giving skills without the benefit of pictures to prompt him.

Language evidence

The assessment usually produces so much information from the child that the assessor will have enough insight into the following aspects of verbal language development to make an initial assessment in all these areas. Usually only a very small proportion of children with non-verbal difficulties have any problems with verbal language as this is usually a great strength of theirs. But any residual difficulties are very obvious:

• grammar – discrepancies in the structure of sentences and use of nouns, adjectives, verbs, pronouns, possessive pronouns, etc.

• continuing issues with regard to articulation

• vocabulary – if his vocabulary skills relating to his favoured topics are strong and those relating to everyday tasks are poor, this will become immediately apparent

• functions of language – distinguishing questions, commands, reporting, etc.

Behaviour

The final area of information gained will be with regard to the child's behaviour when the interpretation levels of the assessment become too great for his skills. It is very easy to see the stages of deterioration in his behaviour and relate them directly to the communicative level of the task being asked of him. As the interpretation becomes more difficult, he may start to:

• fidget with his hands

• wring his hands

- show anxiety in his face

- change the topic of conversation

- get up

- be distracted by something else in the room and start talking about that

- ignore the assessor.

These are all the early signs of confusion and, in the assessment, as soon as any of these signals are seen the task is stopped and the assessor moves on. This is one of the key structures used in the assessment to prevent the build-up to a 'full-blown' behavioural response that will benefit neither the child nor the assessment.

How to set up the assessment

The assessment needs to happen in a quiet room, preferably with a table and two or three chairs. The room should be big enough to have space to video and should not be interrupted by anyone else for the duration of the assessment.

It should be one-to-one. It is possible for one other person to observe but never the parent. This is because the parent (wittingly or otherwise) will have an effect on the child, according to what sort of relationship they have with him. It doesn't matter if this is a good relationship or bad, but the child may look to the parent to speak for him or not say something because he is worried about the parent knowing about it, for example. The child needs the scope to be himself, to speak freely, independently and without influence.

Structured approach

The assessment needs visual prompts to tell the child:

- what is going to happen

- what activity is taking place

- when an activity has finished

- when the end will be.

These are typical prompts used in autistic programmes but are really important for this assessment. This will be the first time that the assessor has met the child and therefore if the assessment is going to achieve what it sets out to, the structure must support the child to communicate with you to the best of his ability.

Using this structure and abandoning the assessment at the first sign of the child going into confusion are the two factors that have helped me assess so many children with severe behavioural difficulties when others would not even contemplate working in such close proximity as is necessary to undertake the assessment.

What you will find on assessment

The assessment is divided into four parts:

1 information-giving. This establishes whether the child understands both shared knowledge and how much information to give to meet the listener's needs.

2 Interpretation of three basic emotions – happy, sad and angry.

3 Observation and interpretation of simple 'what's wrong?' situations.

4 Interpretation of complex information and level of prediction skills.

Mismatch between language and non-verbal communication skills

The assessment will always reveal a mismatch between the child's verbal expressive skills and his non-verbal communication skills. Expressive language skills may well be functioning at his age level or beyond. His non-verbal communication skills may well be functioning below a three-year-old level. Unless this mismatch is addressed, his problems will worsen.

Evidence gained

The Not Just Talking method sets out to assess whether the child:

1 can give good and adequate information without visual clues to prompt him

2 understands high-level basic emotions and can talk about the causes of these emotions in the people in the pictures

3 recognises and can talk about anomalies in information

4 is able to draw conclusions from complex information with three or more people in the scenario and know from this information what is going to happen next in the story.

As an unexpected consequence of the assessment there is a great deal of information about his language skills – articulation, grammar and vocabulary – as well as an insight into how differently he understands language according to the task.

Once all this information is obtained, it is possible to feed back to parents and teachers the areas of communicative difficulty the child has and plan the appropriate level to start the intervention programme.

Many children will have a profile that shows excellent skill use in certain areas, for example, they are able to look at people and give a full level of information about basic emotions. However, any sign of struggling in the assessment should sound warning bells in your head. Only by doing one or two of the intervention sessions will you find out if in fact the child has a more serious difficulty that he has learned to mask effectively enough to perform well in the assessment. So if a child is showing signs of any of the behaviours above, then persevere, even if they perform better than expected in assessment.

Final information

All but two of the children who have participated in the Not Just Talking assessment over the past 15 years have gone on to benefit from the intervention programme.

Case example 1

The first was more than 15 years ago but I will never forget him. Charlie was about 14 and at a moderate learning disability school (the term in those days which often meant that their behaviour was not appropriate for mainstream school.)

His parents had parted and he lived with his dad. I went to assess him and he was in a room on his own because of his behavioural difficulties. When I entered the room, Charlie refused to talk. I used the structures of the assessment and showed him what I was going to do and told him how long it would take, but after 20 minutes he had said nothing.

I left the room and there was a learning support assistant waiting to see how I had got on. When I told her the outcome she said she was not entirely surprised because his father had told him that 'He couldn't talk to women'!

If I had known this before I entered the room I would have planned the session differently, but as it was, there was no possible way that Charlie would have communicated with me. His 'rule', out of a probable selection of a few others, told him that he wasn't able to talk to women and therefore he didn't even try.

Case example 2

The second was a girl, Pauline, who had been wrongly labelled as 'the worst girl in the country'. Because part of the process of the assessment involves getting video evidence of the child's conversational skills, I always advise parents and teachers not to mention this aspect of the assessment.

Also, I rarely tell people what will happen in the assessment. This is because if people then tell the child what is going to happen – even with the best of intentions – the child can only process the information through his limited interpretational skills. His prediction skills will also be poor and may well predict things that he dreads, leading to a breakdown in his behaviour.

Pauline decided to go under the kitchen table and did not come out, screaming and saying some choice words to try to get rid of me!

However, even those children with severe behaviour problems, if they are not given this information, become compliant and cooperative for the half-hour of the assessment. I have had many comments after teachers have seen the film of the assessment that reveal their surprise at how much I was able to get from the children, who tend to give little information in day-to-day situations unless talking about their preferred topics.

Here are a few examples of responses that I have had over the years to questions in the assessment. They can be amusing or completely confusing, but they give an indication of how far the children are from being able to make good sense of what they see:

 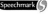 Speechmark Ⓢ

Example 1: limited information-giving (misdirection and distraction)

- *Emily was very poor at giving information at the age of six. If she was unable to tell me what I asked she just said 'I can't remember'. Children who feel that they are unable to give you what you want to hear will make something up or have developed a strategy like this to fob you off – if she can't 'remember' there is nothing much you can do to get her to give the information required on assessment. If it were during the intervention, thowever, you would prompt her to give more information.*

- *Another strategy might be just to get up and talk about something else. Joshua, who was six on assessment, when asked a too-complex question just jumped up and went to the window to identify whether it was a fly or a bee buzzing! Again, he stopped the conversation quite easily, although because I was in assessment mode, I redirected him to the task when he returned.*

- *An autistic boy, John, would jump up where he was, wave his hands in the air and say, 'If you got it right, give yourself a SuperShiny!' This was just a 'learned phrase' from a young children's TV show that John would use whenever he was confused by what people were saying to him. As a five-year-old this was deemed 'cute', but by seven or eight years old it just looks odd to others, particularly peers.*

Example 2: confusing information-giving

- *Sometimes the information-giving was so far from reality that, without verification from a third party who knew what the correct information was, it was hard to know whether what the child said was correct! Jacob had told me that only he and his mum lived at his house:when asked where his dad lived, he said that his dad lived at work.*

- *I have also been told that fathers go to work by aeroplane and that the child has no siblings when he has. This is not about giving the wrong information intentionally; the child is trying hard to give the information requested, but just can't do it and so tells you whatever he can.*

Example 3: poor interpretation

- *Many of the children assessed struggle with the cause of people's feelings: they can't attribute a cause based on the body language or the situational clues. A picture of a man who is very angry is rarely interpreted as being angry because the children tend to look at one aspect of his body language – his eyes.They think that because the background is black that he has been shocked by a ghost! This is extraordinary, since most of the children, especially when they are in their early teens, have seen many people getting very angry with them.*

- *Another reason why they don't identify in the assessment that the man is angry is that they can't hear him. I think that many of the children only recognise that someone is getting very angry with them when they hear that person shouting.*

- *A common problem with the more sophisticated picture in the complex story sequence at the end of the test is that many children interpret the first picture – three people sitting in a waiting room – as them being at home. When asked what makes them think that, they reply, 'There's a carpet and a radiator.' The children are looking at the wrong information to make sense of what is going on. They should look at the body language of the three people to spot that they are sitting in a manner that indicates they are waiting and probably at the doctor's because of the little girl's anxiety level.*

- *Moving on to the next picture, which is a scene in the doctor's surgery, some children do not see the man as a doctor. They hang on to their interpretation that the people are at home and view the man either as the father or a computer trainer who is helping them with the computer. The child often completely ignores the clues that we would use subconsciously – the most obvious one here being the stethoscope round his neck.*

It is easy to see from these results at assessment how people could assume that the child was interpreting the world in the same way as them and was simply being 'naughty' or deliberately confusing.

Assessment of babies

The assessment of babies only takes a few minutes' observation to achieve. Parents or any early years workers, such as health visitors and midwives, could easily do this. In fact, the latter could routinely do a very brief screening assessment to check that the baby is interested in faces. Parents could be asked to record evidence each day of the non-verbal skills in this assessment.

Within the first three months of a child's life, it is fairly easy to establish whether the child can:

- show interest in faces
- share interest in objects
- anticipate activities and people
- give and take within a 'conversation' while feeding
- produce gurgles and coos in response to what is said to him.

Then it would be relatively easy to put in place a programme that ensures that all babies can do these things. Early assessment would lead to more effective communication later in life for all children.

Assessing non-verbal children

With regard to assessment of non-verbal children later in life, ie, over the age of two or three years, this would be an observational assessment as for babies above, associated with information from parents.

Anyone interested in learning to do this and receiving further information about how to do it should contact Not Just Talking: www.notjusttalking.co.uk.

CONCLUSION

Not Just Talking assessments are available for all the following situations:

1 Talking children with behavioural, social, emotional and educational difficulties. This particular assessment could be used as a pre-school or earlier screening tool to eliminate non-verbal problems as early as possible, ie, before the behaviour problems become too great.

2 Pre-talking babies and toddlers.

3 Non-verbal children, including those on the autistic spectrum who may be much older and even teenagers.

Once you have this assessment information you can plan an intervention for the children who are already talking or a support programme for parents and carers for those children who can't talk yet. When the levels of skill and need are identified through the assessment, it is then possible to place a child on the Not Just Talking intervention programme at the point that will best suit their individual profile.

INTERVENTION

12

A child who has not developed the essential non-verbal skills discussed in this book will have no idea how significant this 60–90 per cent of communication is in helping her to understand what is said to her and enabling her to handle conversations more easily. Open this door for her and, once she goes through, she can never come back – nor will she want to. Also, she will sail on all by herself because the skills will accumulate automatically as she holds ever-more effective conversations.

Throughout the intervention you will be trying to develop the child's understanding of what 'generally' happens. Only then will the child learn to understand the exceptions to these rules. For instance, you might say that boys always have their hair cut short round their ears. Later the child will understand that there are variations on this and some have longer hair. But unless the child has this generalised view of boys, she will not be able to differentiate easily and at a glance between the common traits of boys and girls.

■ WHICH CHILDREN WILL BENEFIT?

The beauty of this intervention method is that it can be used with children from when they are really able to talk, ie, from about three to 19 years of age. It is also possible to use the intervention with adults, but only those who are exceptionally well motivated to change their behaviour. I have never used it with adults who have not chosen it as a course of action. It would be wrong to work with an adult and give them these skills in their forties, for example, unless they really wanted to change. It would be like telling them that all their previous life was lived in a state of confusion which could have been put right while they were in primary school.

Here is a summary of a case involving a father I did take on.

Case example: adult intervention

I was approached by a social services department after they had witnessed the benefit of the Not Just Talking intervention with a 14-year-old. She had been diagnosed with 'appositional disorder', which meant she could not relate her current life to her disturbed childhood.

A social worker had been working with her twice a week for an hour each session to try to get her to talk about her childhood. Within the first six sessions of intervention with Not Just Talking, the social worker contacted me, clearly overjoyed. For the first time ever this girl had started to relate her childhood experiences to her current behaviour.

Impressed by this change, they approached me and asked if I would do a trial of working with a whole family. I was wary because of my concerns about opening this door too late for people, but was told that if Geoff, the man in question, didn't change his behaviour he would lose custody of his children. They also were sure he wanted to change. I felt that this was sufficient motivation.

They described his difficulties as mainly having major altercations with his mother, whom he didn't live with, and being very difficult for the social work team to talk to because he just wanted to tell them what was in his mind. He didn't listen to their advice well. He had a reputation for shouting in meetings as well.

I saw Geoff once and talked about the centrality of non-verbal information to our communication and gave him an insight into how this worked. I also gave him the Not Just Talking Strategy© and practised this during the session. I then arranged to see him the following week.

He arrived the next week a bit upset. I asked what was wrong and this is what he said:

> *'I remembered what you said but I was at my mum's house at the weekend, and it was only on the way home in the car that I realised I had misunderstood what she said. I want to be able to do this at the time not half an hour later.'*

I told Geoff that it was really early days and that in due course it would happen all the time while he was talking. We completed the second session but because of time problems, apart from his attendance at two or three sessions to observe my work with his two boys (who also had this communication problem but at earlier and different stages – one was very verbal and the other hadn't started talking yet), I didn't see Geoff again until a few weeks later at the meeting which was to decide whether or not he kept his children.

I was sitting at a huge table in the social services office where there were about 20 other professionals from all areas of this family's life – health, education and social services – all people who would influence the decision about the future of his children. That would be a daunting prospect for most people with good communication skills.

Geoff walked into the room and his social worker started talking to him. I was sitting behind her and after a few moments she turned to me and raised her eyebrows. She couldn't believe the change in him: he was calm and appropriate in his communication with her. He then sat and listened to all the comments by the professionals and waited his turn to talk. When he spoke he was clear but there was no sign of his previous anger. Everyone present was stunned at the change in him. Geoff kept his children as a result.

My contention about the Not Just Talking intervention is that essentially all that's necessary is to open the door and show people that there is more to communication than just the spoken words. If people are bright enough and motivated enough they will pass through the door and use the information on their own. They do not need their hand holding beyond this point.

In fact, I have had difficulty discharging some children, particularly because their parents are so pleased with the intervention that they worry that the child will deteriorate if I stop seeing her. Given the opportunity to continue to develop skills in a variety of different situations, children and adults will do it by themselves. That is how children develop these skills in normal circumstances: we don't focus on them, they pick up the skills from holding and watching conversations.

Who won't benefit?

The only children who will not benefit from this intervention are:

- older children who have boxed themselves in so much that they won't accept the helping hand offered by the intervention

- children who are in a situation where the parents and school believe the child is choosing to talk and behave inappropriately and/or don't believe that the child can improve through the intervention

- those who have a very supportive school but the home situation is not supportive. The intervention can work, but those adults who do support the intervention just need to work a bit harder. It is, of course, understood that all school and social service teams are doing their best to help parents appreciate the needs of their child

- those where there is complete inconsistency of approach. This can happen at home or in schools, for example, if her class teacher is really committed but the girl goes out to play and the playground staff aren't using the strategies, then the child will be held back.

However, never assume that the child won't benefit – it is only after intervention has been attempted that you can make that judgement. Here is a case history recounted to me by someone recently trained in the Not Just Talking intervention techniques:

Case example

The practitioner had been referred a young boy who had been identified as having a possible ADHD diagnosis. Tom was a real handful in the mainstream school as he was unable to settle and as a result was quite disruptive to the other children.

The intervention started and Tom began to blossom. She told me that instead of rushing back to class at the end of their session and disrupting the other children, which was his usual style, after only a couple of sessions he would only need a brief prompt to look for a space to sit in. If he identified that there was none, he would ask appropriately for his classmates to move and make space for him. The class teacher also noticed a real improvement in his independent work skills because his concentration and focus had improved so much. Everyone felt most positive about his academic and social potential.

However, Tom's mother, who was a single parent, found his behaviour hard to deal with at home so took him to a doctor who prescribed medication for hyperactivity. This caused a severe deterioration in his ability to focus and concentrate and the medication was changed a few times as a result. However, nothing helped him return to the pre-medication state. So after starting the medication all the progress he made with the Not Just Talking intervention disappeared. Tom is now likely to leave mainstream school because he has deteriorated academically. Both the person undertaking the intervention and the school feel helpless to do anything to stop this.

Under circumstances such as these, there is little that can be done. Because what happened outside the school situation had such a negative affect on the child and there was no way that the school could change the prescription, he could no longer benefit from the help that the programme had offered. As such, it was deemed that there was no way out of this conundrum.

Only when parents, medics and educationalists all understand the benefits, in terms of behaviour and hyperactivity, of improving non-verbal understanding, will situations of this kind cease. In my experience this story is not unusual, as medication often subdues the child. However, ideally all children should have the opportunity to experience the benefit of intervention before medication is even contemplated. One important advantage of the programme is that intervention will not change the child or her personality – only her communication skills will be improved, allowing her true personality to shine through.

Why the intervention works

The intervention works so well because, once the child has learned the strategies of being a good listener and how to process information, she cannot forget them – they are in her subconscious mind. This is where we all store this huge amount of beneficial experiential knowledge. Each situation in which she communicates is now seen through a new lens. She is no longer looking at all the non-verbal information, which would simply overload her. She can focus in order to make good sense of what she sees and hears. And this positive experience only increases her confidence and drive to improve further.

WHO CAN DO THE INTERVENTION?

There are no prerequisite qualifications for carrying out the intervention. Those with the following characteristics are ideal:

- an open, sunny disposition

- a deep desire to help the child become an independent communicator

- a level of skill, knowledge and experience that will enable them to work effectively with the Not Just Talking programme.

However, there are certain people who will find it harder than others and as such may not be ideal candidates:

- Speech and language therapists: this is only because, in order to be really good at the intervention, you need to forget about language development and trust that the intervention in the long term will improve all these areas of communication. If a speech and language therapist looks at the child from a language perspective rather than through a non-verbal one or tries to improve the child's expressive language by working on her categorisation skills or developing vocabulary in other ways, then these areas will continue to exceed the level of her non-verbal skills and the child won't improve.

- People who cannot let go of the idea that the child is choosing to behave or speak in inappropriate ways may not be able to see the child's confusion for what it is.

- Anyone who wishes to 'mother' the child and protect them. The intervention requires a determination to give the child communicative independence and doing everything for them is contra-indicated.

- Those people who are fixed on behaviourist strategies, such as psychologists or those practising Facilitated Communication and other programmes based on the behaviourist principles of the stimulus–response mechanism for communication.

Why parents can't intervene with their children

Although it is fairly straightforward for parents to change their approaches to their children in order to promote non-verbal communication skills rather than verbal language skills, it is not possible for parents to undertake the intervention with their own children.

The aim of the intervention is to improve the child's communication in all situations and with whoever she wishes to communicate. Parents and children have too much shared knowledge and this creates practical problems in assessing and working with the child's real level of understanding. The child also needs to learn the skills to communicate with a relative stranger so that she can gain confidence that her new-found skill will work whatever situation she is in.

Finally, as all parents know, children will not work in a structured manner for half an hour per week as well with a parent as with an outsider! So the intervention can only be done by a person who doesn't know the child too well. It may also be that a teacher who has a good and strong relationship with the child will not be the best person to undertake the intervention.

THE AIM OF THE NOT JUST TALKING INTERVENTION

Those children who need the intervention will have limited ability to communicate effectively in all situations and may even be 'shut down', ie, not attempting to communicate unless they choose to.

Through the intervention you will enable every child to talk in a suitable manner to whoever they wish to talk to. This will be achieved through improving the following skills:

- Processing all the non-verbal information necessary to make best sense of each situation they find themselves in.

- Ignoring irrelevant visual information that will only confuse them further.

213

- Understanding the role of the listener – which in turn will help them to know what a speaker has to do. This is to keep conversations going for as long as necessary to meet the needs and expectations of the participants in the conversation.

- The ability to give good information, appropriate to the person and situation, without needing to be prompted by others. This is the ultimate goal for the child and will be an indication that they no longer need the intervention.

All these skills will enter the child's subconscious so that they are able to use them at conversational speed as we do all day long. Because the skills enter the subconscious, the child is not able to lose them and therefore is unable to revert to their previous lack of knowledge and skill.

Certain circumstances, such as Christmas or sudden change to timetabling or excessive demands on them academically, socially or emotionally, may affect the child so that they look like they are returning to their previous confused state. However, when those circumstances are resolved, the child will return to the communicative state they had achieved before the change in behaviour. They will not lose the skills they have developed, but you might just need to coax them back into use.

HOW TO STRUCTURE NOT JUST TALKING INTERVENTION SESSIONS

It is important to get the session structure right as recommended. Full information, and examples of the sheets required, will be found in the Not Just Talking Intervention Resource Pack which will be available in 2012. Here you will find out about the types of structures that will be beneficial.

Room requirements

As with the assessment, a quiet room is needed which is not going to be interrupted, preferably without windows as they are a distraction. If there are windows, the therapist should make sure the playground is not outside as other children might distract the child. This is only a significant problem at the start of intervention. Soon the child will be able to cope with interruptions and return to her task appropriately. A table and two chairs will be required.

Visual prompts

These are used at the start of the intervention, to tell the child:

1 what is going to happen

2 how to be a good listener

3 the Not Just Talking interpretation strategy.

These visual prompts should only be used for as long as the child really needs them. The aim of the intervention is to enable the child to be an independent communicator. If she needs to carry around prompt sheets in order to communicate, it may slow her progress to independence.

Most children who have participated in the Not Just Talking intervention have not needed these sheets beyond about the fourth session (and usually before this). Those who need the prompts longer than this are usually on the autistic spectrum or learning disabled.

Who can be present?

During the intervention it is possible for a 'significant other' (apart from parents) to be present. However, I would only recommend this once the therapist is really confident and definitely not for the first session. This confidence comes with increased experience of the intervention programme, and after about six months of regular sessions the therapist will have a strong sense of its effectiveness.

When working with older children with complex conversational difficulties, ie, those who have developed deep strategies to control the conversation and believe their method of communication works for them, it can be very helpful to have a second person in the session to verify interpretation or use as a model for conversation.

The process of an intervention session

The child is asked to sit down and immediately shown the timetable telling her what is going to happen and when the session will end. She is asked what will happen when the session is finished. Usually at the start of intervention the child won't know the answer, but soon she will understand that she is either going back to class or to lunch or out to play. This indicates that her prediction skills are improving.

The therapist then works with the child through the activities for the session. These may be:

1 Face pictures

2 'What's different?' pictures

3 Story sequences

4 Game

5 Finish.

As each activity is finished the child is encouraged to cross it off the list. If she won't, the therapist does it for her until she can do it for herself. The child is given control within the session as soon as possible. She needs to learn that she can control events around her through communication and she doesn't need to resort to behaviour. If things are done for her, she won't learn this important skill.

The resources

The pictures in the Not Just Talking intervention programme have been sorted according to their level of complexity of interpretation. They must be presented in the correct order or the child won't progress as intended.

However, with individual children, a more experienced therapist might use a card two or three ahead in the programme to find out whether the child has jumped a level. I would suggest that to gain this level of experience you need to work with children at least three times a week over a period of 6 to 12 months.

The conversational areas to be addressed

The process of developing interpretation is based on passing over basic understanding of the skill to the child and then developing her ability to a sufficient level for her to do without visual or verbal prompts.

What skills are we talking about here? Put very simply, they are all the skills discussed in the preceding sections. Some develop because you will be working directly on those skills but others evolve as part of the child's increased ability to make better sense of communication situations. She may automatically become better at being a good speaker, her body language might become more expressive or her prediction skills will improve. But if these don't improve as she makes progress in other areas then you will need to work on them specifically. This is why in the intervention programme I tell people how to develop all the skills associated with effective conversations.

Conversation seen as a game of catch

Probably the easiest way of getting across the central part played by the speaker and listener within a conversation is to think of it as a game of catch. This is a good way to get children to understand how a conversation works. The essential elements of are:

1 the thrower (speaker)

2 the ball (message)

3 the catcher (listener).

It is impossible to have a game of catch without all three elements, because there is no game of catch if one element is missing, ie:

- no one to throw the ball

- no ball, or

- no catcher.

The same applies to a conversation – without the speaker, message and listener being present and participating equally there is no conversation.

Also, the way the ball is thrown in a game of catch determines whether the game can proceed and from the table below you will see that the same applies to a conversation:

Game of catch	Conversation
Ball not too high or too low	If the message is too easy or too difficult the listener won't understand
Ball not too slow or too fast	Rate of delivery is important – depending on the situation – for the message to be understood
Ball thrown in awkward or straightforward manner	A message should be as straightforward and clear as the listener and situations dictate
Thrower throws the ball in the wrong direction	Speaker directs the message to the wrong person
Ball is thrown too short or too long	Speaker gives a message that contains too little or too much information for the listener's needs
Thrower doesn't know how to throw	Speaker does not have the skills to be a good speaker
Catcher is not looking at the thrower	Listener is not looking at the speaker and misses the non-verbal clues to help understand the message
Catcher not ready	Speaker not looking so not aware that the listener is not yet ready
Catcher doesn't know how to catch	Listener does not have the skills to be a good listener

The listener's role

Remember that this means what the listener needs to do to make the conversation go better. It does not mean how well the child is listening using auditory discrimination skills, auditory memory and sequencing skills.

The focus of your attention will be determined by the child's skill level. So if she is good at looking at people but can't sit still, focus on getting her to listen. In my experience, at least 95 per cent of my caseload has facial interest as their principal problem area.

First, you need to agree with the child what the listener's role is. Because of all the work done in schools, many children know that they have to listen, but have no idea what that means in reality.

The only way to ensure that a child can look, be still and listen is to demonstrate what it feels like:

1 not to be looked at while being spoken to

2 to have someone wriggling or fidgeting while you are trying to tell them something

3 to have someone respond with a completely different topic from the one you have asked them about.

Once the child has this understanding, you can use it to reinforce good listening technique on those occasions when she doesn't apply it.

The speaker's role

This role often develops naturally following the child's improved ability as a listener. If it doesn't, you should work on:

1 looking at the listener sufficiently

2 being still

3 giving good information.

Because the first two skills are covered in the listener's role, here I am only going to focus on information-giving skills.

One of the main changes in a child during the intervention is that she will learn which information is appropriate to give because she learns to identify and interpret key information regarding who she is talking to and where they are holding the conversation. The transformation from being a child who is only able to focus on what she wants to talk about to a child whose information-giving is suitable whatever situation she finds herself in is a significant step and rewarding to observe.

■ INTERPRETATIONAL SKILLS

Interpretation includes all the skills surrounding the understanding of emotions, body language and situations. Along with developing the listener's role in the child, you will focus all the activities on improving the child's ability to make good sense of what she sees.

This is achieved through getting her to learn by heart the Not Just Talking Interpretation Strategy© available in the intervention guidebook and simply practising it over and over again by looking at pictures which are designed to increase in complexity of interpretation. These picture resources will include:

 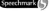

1 single pictures of one or more people showing emotion about something contained in the picture

2 single pictures of people demonstrating something plainly wrong

3 pairs of pictures in which something is different or missing

4 sequences of two or more cards which tell stories about everyday activities.

I have specifically selected pictures of real people doing real things in and outside the home. The Not Just Talking Resource Pack will contain photo cards, all chosen to work from simple to complex interpretation in straightforward steps so that the children experiencing the programme will progress quickly. The whole programme is contained in this resource pack and all you have to do is follow one card with another.

It is not possible to use cards more than once unless the child's interpretational skills are so poor that she doesn't recognise the pictures. Then you can go back over them and promote higher-level interpretation at the same time, something which the child wouldn't have been able to do earlier in the intervention when she first saw the card.

As part of the intervention the child is helped to identify emotions at their different levels, particularly with relation to low, mid and high level expression of emotions. Once the child has recognised these levels she will start to develop the intermediate levels for herself.

Another element of promoting interpretational skills is through looking for information in other good quality pictures such as those in the I Spy... books by Walter Wick (1992–1999). These can also be used to develop conversational skills around sharing information, for instance, 'I have found the duck, can you find the red truck?' These are American books and tend to jump rather sharply between levels of complexity of interpretation. Not Just Talking hopes to publish some similar books with English vocabulary and lower levels of interpretation moving to more complex interpretation in simple steps.

Signs of improvement in interpretation

One of the skills children often lack on entry to the intervention programme is being able to make use of information given to them to help them make better sense of what they see.

When you realise that the child has started doing this, it is a sign of a highly significant breakthrough. The change will be small at the start but suddenly you will realise that instead of arguing that what they were saying is the correct way of seeing things, they will say things like 'Oh yes, I see now' or 'Now it makes sense to me'. Once she demonstrates the ability to read a range of clues effectively, she will be motivated to go further.

ASSOCIATED SKILLS

Cognitive and reasoning skills

Another set of skills that will automatically improve as a result of the intervention method are those associated with prediction, anticipation and drawing conclusions. All the information you request during the half-hour session will be centred around these skills. Although they are often not regarded as conversational skills, the ability to anticipate and to draw conclusions are essential to holding effective conversations.

Choice

It is very easy to assume that a child is choosing, especially if she has learned to say 'yes' as an avoidance tactic for conversations. So give the child many opportunities to choose during the session and remember that a choice is an informed one only if the child knows what happens as a consequence of choosing either option. To develop choice initially you must offer a negative and a positive choice. Once the child can do this, she will move on to being able to select a genuine preference.

Sometimes if the child really finds the initial few sessions difficult, I offer a choice of which order to do the activities.

Identifying options

This is a higher-level skill that will only obviously develop once the child is able to choose. It is the ability to have a selection of options available for each situation you enter and then from that selection choose the most appropriate option.

However, in my experience, it is not usually necessary to work directly on this skill as it automatically occurs as a result of the Not Just Talking intervention programme. So just check that the child is developing these skills and, if not, they will need to be worked on more directly – see the Not Just Talking intervention programme for more information.

Negotiation

One of the purposes of holding conversations is being able to negotiate. Of course, negotiation will only be possible when a high level of conversational skills has developed. Usually a child does not need to be 'taught' how to do this. She will learn from watching others negotiating in many different situations. She will need to observe adults and peers negotiating for different reasons as well, for instance which game to play or how to get out of trouble, so that she can learn these important negotiation skills.

Make sure that people support children by stepping in and modelling how to negotiate if she is struggling to do so or is at risk. Never leave a child to negotiate her own way out of a situation in the playground if you know she has poor conversational skills.

TARGET SETTING

As the intervention makes headway, each session will show either areas of skill that the child needs to develop or areas of progress being achieved. Generally the key targets are developing the listener role and improving interpretational skills using the Not Just Talking Interpretation Strategy. Once these are established, the only targets you will need are related to areas of specific difficulty you uncover, such as:

- a limited ability to recognise age differences

- poor understanding of what people might be thinking

- a lack of vocabulary for everyday tasks such as making the bed or washing up.

Don't be surprised at the speed of progress. Things that you thought the child was unable to do one week may be established by the next. This is why the programme has been proven to deliver positive change within six half-hour sessions.

OUTCOMES

Here are some of the outcomes that you might expect both generally and relating to specific disorders.

Interest in faces

This outcome is the one that starts the whole process of improvement of the child's non-verbal conversational skills. It is central to enabling the child to 'read' information from body language and facial expressions, and to:

- start to understand the meaning of facial expressions and body language

- learn about the different degrees of expressions

- learn the roles of speaker and listener

- understand verbal messages more effectively.

Without this interest in faces, none of the following outcomes will occur. So however long it takes to get a child interested in faces, the benefits are powerful and far reaching.

Body language

Once facial interest is established and the use of the cards is under way, understanding of body language and facial expressions will soon start to follow. Also, once a child starts to learn that there are different feelings and levels of feeling, she will use facial expressions and body language herself more effectively. This is how children develop these skills 'normally', ie, by observing and accumulating knowledge of specific features of body language so that it can be used by the child on other occasions.

Because the intervention is based on 'normal' development, as intervention progresses new skills accumulate according to how well the baseline skills are functioning. This underlying ability level is what she has acquired during her early months of development and you need to be sure that she has this level of skill before expecting her to communicate effectively through spoken language.

Interpretation skills

Improved interpretation of body language will be accompanied by an increase in understanding of new and more complex situations such as the playground or the swimming pool. There will be fewer episodes of confusion and you will no longer need to use the Not Just Talking strategies recommend for dealing with confusion. The child will also recognise different levels of emotion.

Because of the way the Not Just Talking intervention resources are organised, the earliest cards require relatively simple interpretation, gradually increasing in complexity to give the child the skills she needs to be able to interpret information at speed within each conversation she holds.

OTHER SKILLS THAT DEVELOP AS A CONSEQUENCE OF IMPROVED INTERPRETATIONAL SKILLS

As with the improvement in interpretational skills following the development of good facial interest, it is often the case that all the following areas improve incrementally as a consequence of having gained better interpretation skills.

Drawing conclusions

Children who arrive at the intervention either not being able to draw conclusions or only able to describe what they see are soon able to make appropriate inferences based on which they can then predict will happen next. For instance, knowing that people are putting on raincoats and boots in the utility room will allow the child to predict that they are next going out in the rain.

Prediction

A child automatically becomes able to predict as a result of constant practice of the interpretational strategy – to be found in the Not Just Talking Intervention Pack. Soon the child doesn't even have to think about prediction: it begins to occur naturally – as it should.

Change

An improved ability to deal with change is a consequence of having better interpretation and prediction skills. Soon you will find the child is no longer reacting badly to change but instead coping and actually enjoying the experience.

Social rules

Once a child's interpretational skills reach a certain level she will start to pick up 'rules' she observes others following – for instance, standing at an appropriate distance. She will then test this out by applying the rules for herself in similar situations. Soon she will go from having only one or a few rules which she applies in situations – whether or not they are appropriate – to being able to recognise that she has a choice of rules for each situation.

She will also be able to use non-verbal information to decide which rule applies in the circumstance. This automatically builds confidence in the child because she will start to behave in ways that others are expecting and as a result get more positive reactions from them.

Theory of mind

Developing theory of mind is one of the main areas of change that will significantly affect the child's communication and behaviour. It will develop: there is nothing you can do to stop it. A 15-year-old Asperger's lad said this to one of his teachers:

> Before I met Sioban I didn't know what other people were thinking. Now I do, I would rather not know...

The reality was that this lad was getting on so much better with people that there was no way that anyone else wanted him to go back to the grumpy, distracted person he had been.

The minute a child starts to be able to predict what others are thinking, what they are about to say and do, she begins to understand that others can think and feel differently from her – as well as sharing the same thoughts and feelings as her on other occasions. Once she is on this path, there are no limits to the development of her theory of mind.

Generalisation

Children should start to generalise from one situation to another very quickly in the course of the intervention. This is another consequence of improved interpretation skills.

PROSODIC SKILLS

Nursery rhymes

Remember that nursery rhymes are appropriate to use with children up to the age of about 10. If there is a problem with intonation or rhythm, I often choose to use nursery rhymes as the book or game choice at the end of the session. Children with poor non-verbal communication skills are not functioning communicatively at their chronological age level and therefore what is offered by nursery rhymes is often commensurate with the non-verbal communication age.

INTERVENTION SUCCESS

Here is some evidence from the Not Just Talking archive to help demonstrate the effectiveness of the intervention method:

Case history 1

On referral to Not Just Talking, Alfie, aged 14:

- *was struggling to leave the house to go to school because of his anxiety*

- *had no friends at school despite doing really well academically*

- *had been diagnosed with Asperger's syndrome*

- *had received a great deal of support from outreach services but there had been no change in his anxiety levels.*

On assessment, Alfie:

- *was very poor at giving information in a conversation*

- *didn't know what had caused feelings in others*

- *had limited use of non-verbal communication himself*

- *would opt out of situations as a way of dealing with his communication problem.*

Following intervention from Not Just Talking:

- *Alfie's attendance at school improved*

- *he had started to travel on his own into a town 15 miles away on the bus – to his mother's great surprise*

- *he also surprised her by phoning her on his mobile to tell her that he had arrived safely*

- *he was interacting more with his peers and able to tell jokes*

- *he had also gone out with a group from school to buy a leaving present for a teacher – something he would never have done before the intervention*

- *finally, Alfie had started to go to 'Games workshop' sessions on his own. This had been a great interest of his but he had always pursued it on his own at home. Suddenly he began to seek out these sessions and helped in the shop.*

Case history 2

On assessment Karen, aged six, was showing the following symptoms:

- *inexplicable tantrums*

- *interactional difficulties with her siblings*

- *running away in public places, not understanding the impact on her parents despite them telling her how worried they were on many occasions*

- *wanting to dominate her mother because she was unable to deal with other people communicating with her mother, especially her siblings. This meant that she monopolised her mother's attention and other siblings felt jealous and left out.*

The Not Just Talking Assessment demonstrated that Karen:

- *had difficulties with interpreting complex non-verbal information*

- *lacked the ability to initiate conversation appropriately*

- *would answer 'yes' to questions and statements in order to limit her need to participate in the conversation, ie, her strategy for opting out of conversations*

- *was bright but her school felt her interactional difficulties were hampering her educational performance*

- *was very quiet in class – no behavioural problems at school*

- *came over as very shy to most people who didn't understand that this was a symptom of her communication problem.*

After the Not Just Talking intervention, Karen:

- *improved her behaviour at home to the extent that she was able to participate in group tennis coaching sessions, which had been impossible before*

- *became more biddable and stopped running off when out with adults*

- *started to have friends home to play*

- *communicated much more effectively and could initiate conversations more appropriately*

- *still required educational support at primary school for her creative writing skills.*

From thinking that she might need a specialised secondary school, her parents were able to send her to the mainstream school of their choice.

Case history 3

Mohammed, aged 16; difficulties pre-assessment were:

- *problems with inappropriate behaviour in class, such as rushing to get to the same desk for each lesson and pushing others out of the way to achieve this*

- *an inability to interact with his peers at all; as a result he had few friends.*

The school knew he was extremely intelligent and wanted to keep him because he was doing Greek, Latin and Hebrew at A level and was predicted to get straight As and A*s, but if his interaction with teachers and peers did not improve they would have to exclude him.

The Not Just Talking assessment demonstrated that Mohammed:

- *dominated conversations*

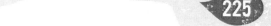

- *was virtually unable to interpret non-verbal information because he was so fixated on the verbal language*

- *was unaware of the roles of the speaker and listener within the conversation*

- *only wanted to tell you what he knew and to demonstrate how clever he was (this did not go down too well with peers)*

- *was unaware of the impact of his behaviour on others.*

When giving information he was so intelligent that he could move the conversation gradually away from the actual topic by a series of complex moves. By the time the listener realised what had happened they were about 10 steps away from the original topic.

During the intervention:

This was one of the most difficult cases that I ever met.

Because I only had six sessions to make a difference with him, his form tutor sat in on the sessions.

Mohammed was so intelligent that he had an answer to everything and refused to countenance that what we were doing in our subconscious was to process the non-verbal information available. By the fourth session, I was beginning to think that this was to be the first 'failure' of the Not Just Talking method.

The session lasted much longer than the allotted half an hour and he totally confused the pair of us so that in the evening I phoned his tutor to debrief. Neither of us really knew how he got to the topic and explanation for his belief that there was no 'non-verbal story' behind the words. So I thought that I should just get on with the last two sessions and hope there would be a change.

However, at the next session it was like a light had been turned on in his brain. He suddenly 'got' that there was non-verbal information and because he was so intelligent he applied it almost immediately!

This is what his tutor said: 'I couldn't believe my eyes when I walked into the form room: he was standing by the radiator watching some other boys who were playing a game of cards. Not only that but he was engaging with them about the card game!' She couldn't believe the change in Mohammed's demeanour

After the Not Just Talking intervention:

- *he continued to progress*

- *there were far fewer problems around the school and with teachers*

- *he stayed at the school and got all his A levels*

- *he went to one of the top universities in the country.*

CONCLUSION

This has of necessity been a simple overview of the Not Just Talking intervention methods and their positive effects. The full Not Just Talking Resource Pack will be available for purchase soon.

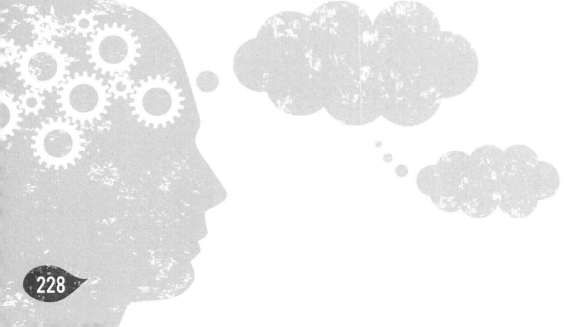

'SHINING THROUGH: THE NOT JUST TALKING APPROACHES'

TRAINING

13

In this last section I will describe the training opportunities that exist for people to work with children's non-verbal communication development difficulties. These are all adjusted for specific needs of the group attending Not Just Talking Training, e.g. people who work with teenagers will have a slightly different awareness-raising training than a cohort who work with primary school children, or prevention training that is for parents of newborn babies compared with training for parents who have had difficulties identified but whose child is lacking non-verbal communication skills.

PREVENTION TRAINING

Not Just Talking: Helping Your Baby Communicate – From Day One

This book is specifically aimed at parents of new babies and gives tips on all the things that parents should do to ensure that their baby develops these non-verbal communication skills.

It also forms the basis of the prevention training programme currently offered by Not Just Talking. By following the main chapter themes, it is possible for any early years professional to use this book as a basis to support parents, either one-to-one or in small groups of not more than 10.

The main elements in the NJT parent training are:

1   A modern malady – where the problem comes from

2   What will happen if a baby fails to develop non-verbal communication skills

3   How to make sure your baby has all these skills

4   How the skills develop

5   The first 24 hours – interest in faces, with video of babies showing these skills (See figure 1 below)

6   What is my baby trying to tell me?

7   The benefits of structure and routine

8   How to help baby give and take communicatively

9   How to promote prediction

10 Tips on promoting communication skills through feeding

11 How the baby makes sense of the world

12 The impact of baby equipment and how to resolve this

13 How to build self-awareness

14 Using nursery rhymes to promote non-verbal skills

15 How to promote imitation and choosing

16 Use of toys and games to promote communication

17 Early use of verbal skills – the development of language

18 The benefits of eating as a family

19 Helping baby to understand signs

20 Coping with change

21 Baby starts using signing

22 Getting ready to talk

23 How to talk to your baby promoting understanding and expression

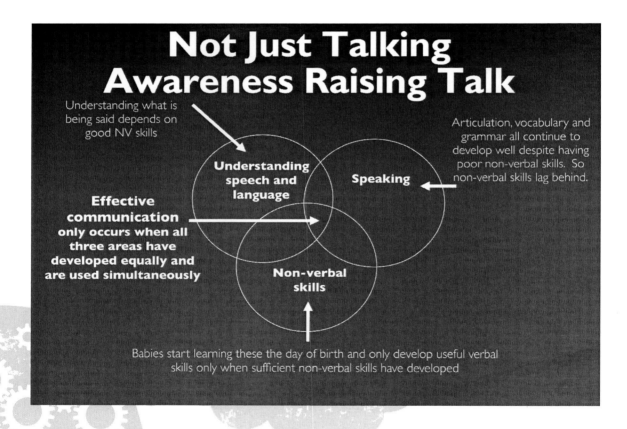

Not Just Talking can train parents, midwives, paediatric nurses, health visitors, social workers and any other early years workers to identify difficulties and promote the missing skills in babies and toddlers.

This training is available for parents and early years specialists. The latter group are able to then use this training with the support of the Not Just Talking parent books, to help

 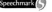

parents promote these skills. If you would like to know more about this prevention training, please contact Not Just Talking – www.notjusttalking.co.uk.

Prevention of communication problems in associated disorders

It is possible to identify children who are at risk of autistic spectrum diagnosis and using the Not Just Talking prevention techniques will ensure that these children are better able to communicate effectively and live lives that are more fulfilled as a result.

AWARENESS-RAISING TRAINING

This is an introduction to where the non-verbal communication problem begins and is necessary for people who have not read this book and who wish to attend the intervention training.

The main elements in the Not Just Talking awareness-raising training are:

1 What are non-verbal communication skills?

2 How do they help communication?

3 Workshop 1 – coping with poor conversational skills

4 What happens to children who fail to develop these skills?

5 Problems faced by families and those working with the children

6 Workshop 2 – coping with poor interpretational skills

7 Strategies to use and those to avoid

8 Evidence of NJT intervention success

Those who read this book will gain much of this information but will not have the experience of the workshops or see the videos of the intervention.

Changing attitudes

What this training (or reading this book) offers is a chance to look at the child in a different way for those working and living with children who demonstrate behaviour problems. They will see the child as not choosing his behaviour but actually as someone in a state of confusion. Once this shift is made, participants are able to empathise more effectively with the child and support their communication rather than hinder it. As a result, everyone has a more positive attitude to the child and his communication.

INTERVENTION TRAINING

This is available from Not Just Talking for anyone who works with children and has some experience of one-to-one sessions. When the Not Just Talking Resources become available from Speechmark Ltd, schools and health teams will be able to purchase these and start the intervention programme. However, if support is required this can be purchased from Not Just Talking.

ASSESSMENT TRAINING

Assessment training is only available to those professionals who are already trained to do assessments. This is because the Not Just Talking assessment training does not train people in the assessment techniques necessary to make the assessment valid and achieve an objective analysis of what the child can and cannot do.

To undertake the Not Just Talking assessment training, participants need to have had some prior training and experience in assessing children's developmental problems. The programme provides a specific method of identifying the child's capabilities with regard to non-verbal communication but does not teach standard assessment techniques.

The assessment training covers the following areas:

1 What you will be assessing

2 The aims of the assessment

3 The assessment criteria, guidelines, process

4 How to use record the assessment on video

5 Recording and feedback of assessment results

6 Producing notes and plans for intervention from the assessment video

7 Reporting

Again, if you are interested in pursuing this option, please contact Not Just Talking.

CONCLUSION

This section has outlined the range of training options based on Not Just Talking techniques. There will be much more information about the content of and support for training in the Not Just Talking Intervention Resources Pack and the Assessment Pack.

If you would like to know more about any of this training, please contact Not Just Talking – www.notjusttalking.co.uk.

REFERENCES

Alcock V (1988) *The Monster Garden*, Lion Books.

Almond D (1998) *Skellig, Hodder*.

Baby It's You (1994), Channel 4.

Baron-Cohen S (2003) *The Essential Difference: Men, Women and the Extreme Male Brain*, Allen Lane.

Baron-Cohen S, Leslie AM & Frith U (1985) 'Does the autistic child have a "theory of mind"?', *Cognition*, 21, pp37–46.

Booth J (2010) 'Pressure grows over James Bulger killer as Jack Straw keeps silent', *Times Online*, 3 March, www.timesonline.co.uk/tol/news/uk/crime/article7048044.ece (accessed August 2011).

Boyce S (2009) *Not Just Talking: Helping Your Baby Communicate – From Day One*, Not Just Talking.

Cambridgeshire Community Services (undated) 'Speech, Language and Communication Services', www.slc.cambridgeshire.nhs.uk (accessed July 2011).

Farroni T, Menon E, Rigato S & Johnson MH (2007) 'The perception of facial expressions in newborn babies', Reid VM, Striano T & Koops W (eds) *Social Cognition during Infancy, Psychology Press*.

Geary J (2011) I is an Other, Harper.

Gladwell M (2005) *Blink: The Power of Thinking Without Thinking*, Penguin.

Goleman D (1999) *Working with Emotional Intelligence*, Bloomsbury Publishing.

Grobel R (2002) *Splish Splash*, Scholastic Books.

Guettier B (2004) *In the Jungle*, Zero to Ten.

Heath A & Bainbridge N (2000) *Baby Massage*, Dorling Kindersley.

Hello (2011) www.hello.org.uk/ (accessed July 2011).

Hobson P (2002) *The Cradle of Thought*, Macmillan.

Hogg T (2001) *The Secrets of the Baby Whisperer*, Vermilion.

HSBC (2002) 'Cultural differences – an introduction', www.youtube.com/watch?v=JK_NinOmFWw (accessed July 2011).

Jackson L (2003) *Freaks, Geeks and Asperger Syndrome: A User Guide to Adolescence*, Jessica Kingsley.

Kanner L (1943) 'Autistic disturbances of affective contact', *Nervous Child*, 2, pp217–50.

Leslie A (1987) 'Pretense and representation: the origins of "theory of mind"', *Psychological Review*, 94 (4), pp412–26.

Mehrabian A (2007) *Non-verbal Communication*, Transaction Publishers.

Miller M (1998) *Baby Faces*, Simon & Schuster.

Morris D (1997) *Manwatching*, Triad.

Morris D (1969) *The Naked Ape*, Corgi.

Palmer S (2006) T*oxic Childhood*, Orion Health.

Ramsey-Rennels JL & Langlois JH (2007) 'How infants perceive and process faces', Slater A & Lewis M (eds) Introduction to Infant Development, Oxford University Press.

Skynner R & Cleese J (1993) *Families and How to Survive Them, Cedar Books*.

Wick W (1992–1999) *I Spy series*, Scholastic Books

Wick W (2002–2010) *Can You See What I See? series*, Scholastic Books

Williams S & Beck I (1987) *Round and Round the Garden: Play Rhymes for Young Children*, Oxford University Press.

Yell Group (2003) 'Haircut', www.youtube.com/watch?v=_Zyax-iZBk8 (accessed July 2011).